The Bromp
Hospital Gu
Chest Physi

89 class

The Brompton Hospital Guide to Chest Physiotherapy

Barbara A. Webber MCSP

Fifth Edition

Blackwell Scientific Publications

OXFORD LONDON EDINBURGH

BOSTON PALO ALTO MELBOURNE

© The Brompton Hospital 1973, 1977, 1980, 1988

Published by
Blackwell Scientific Publications
Editorial offices:
Osney Mead, Oxford OX2 0EL
  (*Orders*: Tel. 0865-240201)
8 John Street, London WC1N 2ES
23 Ainslie Place, Edinburgh EH3 6AJ
3 Cambridge Center,
  Suite 208, Cambridge,
  Massachusetts 02142, USA
667 Lytton Avenue, Palo Alto
  California 94301, USA
107 Barry Street, Carlton
  Victoria 3053, Australia

First published as *Physiotherapy for Medical and
Surgical Thoracic Conditions* 1960
Revised reprints 1962, 1964, 1967
Second edition (under present title by
D.V. Gaskell and B.A. Webber) 1973
Revised reprint 1974
Reprinted 1975
Third edition 1977
Reprinted 1979
Fourth edition (revised by B.A. Webber) 1980
Reprinted 1982
Fifth edition 1988

Set by Cotswold Typesetting Ltd
Printed and bound in Great Britain
by Redwood Burn of Trowbridge

DISTRIBUTORS

USA
  Year Book Medical Publishers
  200 North LaSalle Street,
  Chicago, Illinois 60601
  (*Orders*: Tel. 312-726-9733)

Canada
  The C.V. Mosby Company
  5240 Finch Avenue East
  Scarborough, Ontario
  (*Orders*: Tel. 416-298-1588)

Australia
  Blackwell Scientific Publications
  (Australia) Pty Ltd
  107 Barry Street
  Carlton, Victoria 3053
  (*Orders*: Tel. 03-347-0300)

British Library
Cataloguing in Publication Data

Webber, B.A.
  The Brompton Hospital guide to chest
  physiotherapy.—5th ed.
  1. Chest   2. Physical therapy
  I. Title   II. Gaskell, D.V.
  617′.54062   RC731

  ISBN 0-632-01978-6

Contents

Preface to fifth edition

The new edition of this practical guide to chest physiotherapy includes many changes and additions throughout the text to keep pace with recent advances and changes in treatment methods and equipment available for the care of cardiorespiratory patients.

A new chapter on paediatrics explains briefly the development of the respiratory system in the infant and differences in the treatment of infants, children and adults. Assessment of the child is emphasized, physiotherapy techniques are discussed and the treatments of specific medical and surgical conditions are outlined.

In an enlarged chapter on adjuncts to physiotherapy the uses of periodic continuous positive airway pressure, glossopharyngeal breathing and minitracheotomy have been added.

This book is intended for students and qualified physiotherapists working in respiratory care and should be used with a background knowledge of anatomy, physiology and pathology gained from specialized texts.

References to support current medical treatment and physiotherapy are included throughout the text. These will help readers to further evaluate and broaden their knowledge on subjects of special interest.

Throughout the text, the pronoun 'he' is used for the patient, while the pronoun 'she' is used for the physiotherapist. This is not intended to imply that all patients are male, or that all physiotherapists are female. I hope that the reader will not be offended by what has been adopted simply as an economical linguistic convention.

I would like to thank Miss Anita Davis for her advice with the surgical section, Mrs Valerie Edmondson with the paediatric section, and Miss Diana Gaskell and my medical colleagues for their helpful comments. I am particularly grateful to Miss Jennifer Pryor without whose enthusiasm and help this new edition would not have been completed.

My gratitude is due to Diana Gaskell for her part as co-author of our first two editions of this book. I am indebted to her for the opportunity of working with her and learning from her wealth of clinical experience.

I would also liked to acknowledge the pioneering work of Miss Gaskell's predecessors, Miss Winifred Linton and Miss Jocelyn Reed, who laid the foundation for respiratory physiotherapy at the Brompton Hospital.

B.A. Webber 1987

vii

Preface to second edition

This book is intended as a practical guide for physiotherapists and others concerned with the treatment of chest conditions. It is derived from the booklet *Physiotherapy for Medical and Surgical Thoracic Conditions* originally compiled at the Brompton Hospital in 1960.

The development of physiotherapeutic techniques in the treatment of chest disease was begun at the Brompton Hospital in 1934 by the late Miss Winifred Linton, FCSP(HON), who became superintendent physiotherapist at that time. These techniques have subsequently been further developed and modified as advances in the medical and surgical management of chest disease have occurred, and more understanding of the physiology of normal respiration has been gained.

The basic techniques of breathing exercises and postural drainage and an outline of the relevant anatomy are described. Physiotherapy for a wide variety of medical and surgical cardio-thoracic conditions is included. There are also sections on the treatment of patients undergoing artifical ventilation and an account of the uses of intermittent positive pressure breathing as a valuable adjunct to physiotherapy.

In order to make intelligent use of the techniques described in the following text, the physiotherapist must have a detailed knowledge of the anatomical mechanism of respiration and the physiology of gaseous exchange. A basic knowledge of the interpretation of electrocardiographs is also useful. This additional knowledge can be obtained from the appropriate text books.

It is important to appreciate that the physiotherapist is a member of a team which includes nurses, technicians and the patient, all under the direction of a physician or surgeon. The more each person is cognisant of the others' contribution, and the more their efforts are co-ordinated, the better will be the results.

The authors would like to thank Dr M.A. Branthwaite MRCP, FFARCS, for assistance and advice given during the preparation of this book. They are also grateful to Professor R.J. Last FRCS, and to Mrs S.A. Hyde MCSP, for their helpful suggestions.

D.V. Gaskell
B.A. Webber

1 Anatomy of the thoracic cage and lungs

MOVEMENTS OF THE RIB CAGE

An understanding of the normal mechanism of respiration is essential before teaching breathing exercises. This mechanism depends not only on the anatomy of the respiratory muscles, but in particular the ribs and their articulations in the thoracic cage. To quote Professor R.J. Last (1972): 'The ribs are to breathe with'.

During respiration changes in volume of the thoracic cage are brought about in 3 diameters:

The antero-posterior diameter of the thorax is increased by elevation of the ribs. The manubrium of the sternum is fixed by a primary cartilaginous joint to the first costal cartilage and the manubrium and the first ribs are fixed to each other and move together as one. As the manubrium is elevated its lower border projects anteriorly. This border articulates by a hinge joint to the body of the sternum, movement occurring at this joint as the body of the sternum rises with the ribs. (If this joint becomes ankylosed, thoracic expansion is virtually lost.)

The costal cartilages of the 2nd to 7th ribs articulate with the sternum by a synovial joint and the 8th, 9th and 10th costal cartilages articulate with the cartilage above by a synovial joint.

The ribs slope downwards from their attachment to the vertebral column towards the sternum, at an angle of 45°. Rotation of the neck of the ribs occurs at all 12 costovertebral joints and this results in elevation or depression of the anterior ends of the ribs.

As a result of the obliquity of the ribs, elevation of the sternum carries it forward and the antero-posterior diameter of the thorax is increased. This up and down movement of the body of the sternum and the ribs attached to it is often termed the 'pump-handle' movement.

The transverse diameter of the thorax is increased in two ways, one passive and the other active. The passive increase is due to the shape of the ribs and the axis round which they hinge during inspiration. The axis is not transverse across the body, but passes through the head and tubercle of each rib obliquely backwards from the midline (figs 1 & 2). Therefore the downward sloping rib is not only elevated antero-posteriorly, but also laterally. This lateral spread of the ribs increases from the 5th rib downwards because the costal cartilages become progressively more oblique. It does not occur in the upper 4 pairs, as their costal cartilages are too short to allow such separation from the midline.

The active increase in transverse diameter is brought about by the 'bucket-handle' movement of the lower ribs. These ribs rotate about an axis that passes

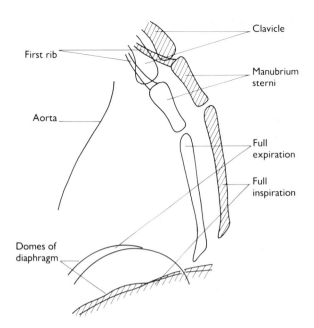

First rib

Clavicle

Aorta

Manubrium sterni

Full expiration

Full inspiration

Domes of diaphragm

Fig. 1. *Lateral X-ray view of the thoracic cavity of a healthy young male, showing maximum excursion simultaneously of the chest wall and of the diaphragm. From R.J. Last (1972).*

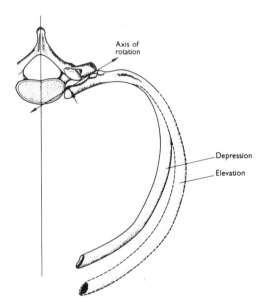

Axis of rotation

Depression

Elevation

Fig. 2. *The axis of rotation of a rib. From R.J. Last (1972).*

through the anterior and posterior extremity of each, like lifting up the fallen handle from the side of a bucket.

This movement can occur because the articular surfaces of the 7th to 10th costo-vertebral joints are flat. The tubercles of these ribs can move up and down in addition to the rotation occurring at the neck of the rib.

The vertical diameter of the thorax is increased by descent of the diaphragm.

THE RESPIRATORY MUSCLES

The respiratory muscles comprise the diaphragm, the intercostals, the scalenes, the abdominals and the accessory muscles. They are either prime movers or they act to stabilize the rib cage and facilitate the action of other muscles. During inspiration the integrated action of the respiratory muscles enlarges the thoracic cavity, negative intrapleural pressure is created and the lungs inflate (Morgan *et al.* 1986).

The diaphragm is bi-domed and is the most important muscle of inspiration. It is largely responsible for quiet breathing with the other muscles acting to stabilize the rib cage. The costal part of the diaphragm arises from the lower 6 ribs and cartilages and runs upwards and parallel to the rib cage before inserting into the central tendon. This lies at the level of the lower end of the sternum during quiet breathing. The crural part of the diaphragm arises from the 2nd to 4th lumbar vertebrae and its associated ligaments and also inserts into the central tendon. When the diaphragm contracts the muscle fibres in apposition to the rib cage shorten, lifting the rib cage and flattening the dome (Green & Moxham 1985).

The diaphragm's inspiratory action depends on its configuration and the presence of abdominal resistance to produce expansion of the rib cage. The higher the dome of the diaphragm the greater the force of contraction. When the diaphragm is flattened as in the pulmonary hyperinflation of emphysema or severe asthma, its inspiratory action is considerably less and it may have an expiratory action.

The intercostal muscles expand or contract the rib cage and provide tone and stability to the intercostal spaces to allow the changes in intrapleural pressure. The external intercostal muscles pass obliquely downwards and forwards and the internal intercostals pass downwards and backwards. Both groups of intercostals have inspiratory activity at low lung volumes and expiratory activity at high lung volumes (De Troyer *et al.* 1983).

The scalene muscles contribute to lift, expand and stabilize the upper rib cage during quiet breathing (De Troyer & Estenne 1984).

The abdominal muscles are predominantly muscles of expiration especially at high levels of ventilation and during coughing, but they facilitate inspiration by maintaining the curvature of the diaphragm (Green & Moxham 1985).

The accessory muscles have inspiratory activity at high levels of ventilation and in respiratory failure. The sternomastoids together with the scalene muscles elevate the thoracic inlet while the head extensor muscles fix the head in extension. If the arms are fixed in abduction, the muscles attaching the upper limbs to the trunk are inspiratory. These are the pectoral muscles, serratus anterior and the costal fibres of latissimus dorsi.

STRUCTURE OF AIRWAYS AND ALVEOLI

It is not intended to give a detailed description of the anatomy and physiology of the respiratory system, but a few facts concerning the structure of the airways are described to assist the understanding of some mechanisms involved in respiratory physiotherapy.

The *trachea* extends from the cricoid cartilage (lower border of C6) to the bifurcation of the main bronchi at the level of the angle of Louis (upper border of T5). It is lined by ciliated columnar epithelium containing plentiful mucus secreting glands and goblet cells. The wall is a fibro-elastic membrane whose patency is maintained by C-shaped rings of cartilage. The gaps lie posteriorly and are closed by a sheet of muscle which plays an important part in the efficacy of coughing and huffing.

The *bronchi* are airways which have cartilage in their walls. The proximal 5 generations have abundant cartilage, but the 5th to 15th generations are smaller bronchi with scattered plates of cartilage throughout the walls. The walls of the bronchi also contain fibrous tissue with a capillary network and longitudinal bands of elastic fibres. They are lined by layers of epithelium containing numerous mucus secreting glands, goblet cells and ciliated cells.

Bronchioli are airways distal to the last plate of cartilage and proximal to the alveolar region. They are about 1 mm or less in diameter. Their walls are composed of smooth muscle fibres arranged circularly and lined by epithelium containing some mucus glands, goblet cells and ciliated cells. The distal bronchioli are lined with one layer of epithelium only

3

and have very few mucus secreting cells.

In massive collapse of a lobe the large bronchi are inherently rigid enough to remain patent, whereas the walls of the small bronchi and bronchioli collapse and come into apposition.

All bronchioli eventually reach a point where alveoli open into the lumen. This part is known as the *respiratory bronchiole*. *Ciliated cells* appear in the epithelial lining of the airways from the level of the respiratory bronchiole and are responsible for shifting mucus and other particles from this level to the larynx. The cilia beat in a liquid layer known as the periciliary layer and the viscous secretions that make up sputum rest on the surface of this liquid (fig. 3). When a patient is dehydrated, the periciliary layer becomes reduced or absent and the cilia become entangled in the mucus, making the clearance mechanism ineffective. A *terminal bronchiole* is defined as the airway immediately proximal to the respiratory bron-

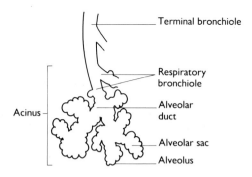

Fig. 4. *Respiratory bronchiole.*

chiole (fig. 4). The terminal bronchioli contain no cilia and no mucus secreting glands or goblet cells.

An *acinus* is the area of lung distal to the terminal bronchiole and includes several generations of respiratory bronchioli (up to 8), alveolar ducts and alveoli. An acinus is approximately 0.5–1 cm in diameter.

An estimate of the total number of alveoli in the average adult lung is in the region of 300 million.

An *alveolus* is an air sac consisting of a single layer of flat cells and a network of fine elastic fibres. A rich network of capillaries surrounds it.

Alveolar pores, known as the pores of Kohn, are openings that exist in the alveolar walls allowing drift of air between adjacent alveoli. This phenomenon of *collateral ventilation*, or collateral air drift also takes place through two other pathways: the canals of Lambert connecting respiratory bronchioles and terminal bronchioles to alveoli and alveolar ducts and the interbronchiolar channels of Martin between respiratory bronchioles (Menkes & Traystman 1977) (fig. 5). Collapse of the lung distal to a plugged bronchus may be prevented by the passage of air through these alternative path-

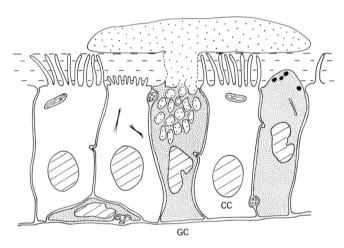

Fig. 3. *Diagrammatic representation of cells in lining epithelium, fluid layer in which cilia beat, and thick mucus that may be on tips of cilia. GC: goblet cell; CC: ciliated cell. By courtesy of Professor Lynne Reid (1973).*

4

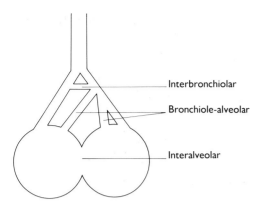

Interbronchiolar

Bronchiole-alveolar

Interalveolar

Fig. 5. *Pathways for collateral ventilation.*

ways. The pleura prevents drift of air between the lobes of the lungs.

Collateral ventilation is less effective in infants and children than in adults because these connections are not fully developed until several years after birth.

With the exception of the alveoli adjacent to the pleura, all the alveoli are surrounded by other alveoli and therefore are supported by each other. This support offered to alveoli by those surrounding them is known as *interdependence* (Mead *et al.* 1970). It has been shown that if a group of alveoli have a tendency to collapse, the surrounding expanded lung tissue produces expanding forces on the collapsed portion. Interdependence may play an important part in the prevention of atelectasis and in opening up areas of collapse.

2 Chest radiographs— basic interpretation

Interpretation of the radiograph is an important part of the assessment of chest disease and although the physiotherapist will depend on the medical staff to interpret the finer details, a basic understanding is valuable.

The radiograph is a photographic negative where the degree of blackening depends on the amount of absorption of X-rays by the structures in their passage. The more solid structures such as bone, fluid and soft tissues absorb more of the X-rays and appear relatively white, while the less solid structures containing air appear relatively black.

The radiograph should always be examined systematically to avoid missing useful information.

POSTERO-ANTERIOR OR ANTERO-POSTERIOR VIEW

In the postero-anterior (PA) or antero-posterior (AP) film the following details are observed:

1 The *name, sex* of the patient and *date* of the film.

2 *Positioning.* The patient should be positioned centrally in relation to the film. If accurately centred, the distance between the medial end of each clavicle and the lateral edge of the vertebral body over which it lies should be equal. Alternatively the distance of the medial ends of the clavicles from the manubrium should be equal. Inequality of this distance denotes rotation of the patient and can lead to misinterpretation of the film.

3 *Exposure.* It is important that the film is neither over nor under exposed. The outline of the vertebral bodies should be just visible through the central mediastinal shadow. It is often useful to compare a recent radiograph with previous films, but differences in exposure must be taken into account.

4 *Soft tissue shadows.* Breast shadows may obscure the lower lung zones. The unilateral absence of breast shadow resulting from mastectomy can be noted. Subcutaneous (surgical) emphysema may be seen as darker areas in between layers of connective tissue in the chest wall. These must not be confused with fat lines. Post-operatively the subcutaneous emphysema may track along the fascial planes outlining the pectoral muscles and neurovascular bundles in the axilla. If the air leaks into the mediastinum, it may seep up into the neck.

It is important that external articles such as dressings, electrodes or an oxygen mask and tubing should not be misinterpreted as intrathoracic shadows.

5 *Bony structures.* The rib cage and spinal column are observed for deformity, the presence of cervical rib, rib fractures and previous rib resection for thoracotomy. Notching of ribs is characteristic of coarctation of the aorta.

Osteoporosis of the bony structures should also be noted. The ribs normally slope symmetrically downwards and forwards from the vertebral column. In scoliosis they slope more steeply on the side of the concavity. Apart from spinal deformity, steeply sloping ribs with narrowed intercostal spaces indicate diminished lung volume on that side from old or recent disease.

The ribs are more horizontal than normal and the intercostal spaces widened when the chest is hyperinflated as in emphysema, asthma or with large pleural effusions.

6 *Trachea.* The shadow of the trachea normally lies centrally with the lower third deviating slightly to the right. Provided the patient has been positioned centrally, any greater deviation of the trachea is helpful in assessing mediastinal shift.

7 *Heart shadow.* The heart shadow is observed for abnormality of outline and 'true' enlargement.

The transverse diameter of the heart is normally less than 50% of the total transverse diameter of the rib cage. In the standard postero-anterior film the patient stands facing and close to the film and the shadow of the heart is approximately the true size. In an antero-posterior film, taken when the patient is confined to bed, the film is placed behind the patient and heart size becomes exaggerated due to geometrical magnification.

In the majority of normal persons, one-third of the heart lies to the right of the midline and two-thirds to the left, but one-quarter to three-quarters is accepted as normal. In emphysema, the heart tends to be narrow and vertical partly as a result of the low position of the diaphragm.

8 *The diaphragm and costo-phrenic angles.*

The two hemidiaphragms should be rounded, smooth, sharply defined shadows with the level of the right dome being normally 2 cm higher than the left in all phases of respiration. If there is a large amount of gas in the stomach or colon, the left dome may be elevated. On a radiograph taken in full inspiration the right hemidiaphragm is intersected by the shadow of the anterior part of the 6th rib (fig. 6a).

In emphysema the domes of the diaphragm are typically low and flattened. The diaphragm is considered low if it is below the anterior end of the right 6th intercostal space. Elevation of one dome of the diaphragm may result from damage to the phrenic nerve or to the muscle itself, or from compression of lung, for example by pleural fibrosis. In the normal radiograph the costophrenic angles should be acute, sharply defined and symmetrical.

9 *Hilar shadows.* The areas of increased density in the medial part of the central portion of the lung fields are known as the hilar shadows. They consist mainly of the pulmonary arteries, their branches and the pulmonary veins. The pulmonary vessels visible throughout the lung fields fan out from the hila. In a normal radiograph the left hilum is obscured by the main pulmonary artery and it lies at a slightly higher level than the right hilum.

Enlargement of both hila is seen when diffuse pulmonary disease leads to an increase in pulmonary artery pressure and also when there is bilateral hilar lymph node enlargement as in sarcoidosis. Enlargement of one hilum is suspicious of malignant disease. Elevation of one or both hila can result from apical fibrosis and unilateral depression of the hilum is associated with collapse of the lower lobe.

10 *Lung fields.* The upper, middle and

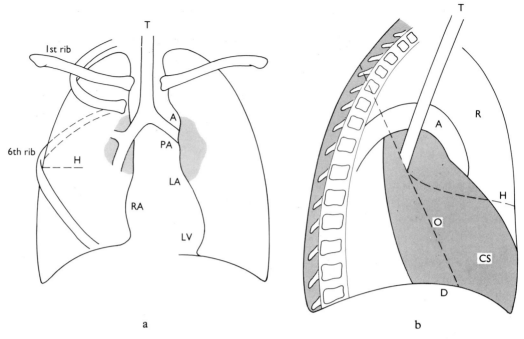

Fig. 6. *Diagram of anatomical features on a normal chest radiograph: (a) PA and (b) lateral views. T: trachea; A: aorta; PA: pulmonary artery; LA: left atrial appendage; LV: left ventricle; RA: right atrium; D: diaphragm; H: horizontal fissure; O: oblique fissure; R: retrosternal air space; CS: cardiac shadow.*

lower zones of the lung fields are compared, one side with the other, for any difference in shadowing. In a normal radiograph the lung markings which are produced by the pulmonary vessels extend over the entire lung fields to the rib cage. Valuable information can be obtained from study of the vessels in the lungs. In the upright position the size of the blood vessels is normally greater in the lower half of the lung than the upper half.

Absence or diminution of the peripheral markings are important signs in emphysema. The habit of scanning the lung vessels from the periphery towards the hilum, helps to concentrate attention on any avascular areas such as pneumothorax at the periphery, or bullae within the lung field.

The bronchi are not usually visible beyond 2–3 cm from the hilum on a normal radiograph unless they are viewed end-on. A bronchus is then seen as a ring-like area of increased density with a central translucency, whereas a blood vessel seen end-on appears as a round solid shadow. This is distinguished from an intrapulmonary nodule by identification of the vessel leading into and out of the opacity.

When the bronchial walls are grossly thickened with disease and if they are also dilated as in bronchiectasis, they may be seen as parallel line shadows.

The horizontal fissure which divides the right upper lobe from the middle lobe is seen in 50–60% of normal persons as a fine hair-like line, at the level of the 6th rib

8

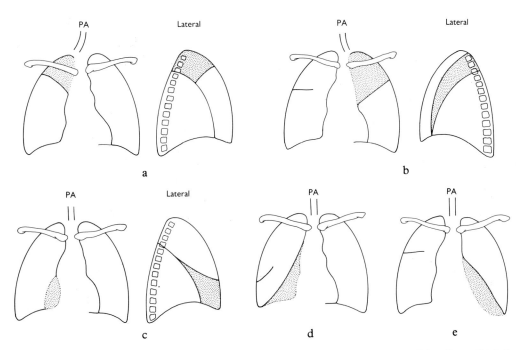

Fig. 7. *Diagrammatic representation of lobar collapse seen on radiographs. (a) Right upper lobe collapse. (b) Left upper lobe collapse. (c) Middle lobe collapse. (d) Right lower lobe collapse. (e) Left lower lobe collapse.*

in the mid-axillary line, extending horizontally to the level of the 3rd or 4th costal cartilage anteriorly. In the normal the outer end may curve slightly downwards. Deviation of this fissure is a guide to shrinkage of the right lung resulting from lobar collapse or fibrosis (fig. 7). The right and left oblique fissures are not normally visible on the postero-anterior film.

LATERAL VIEW

A lateral chest radiograph is helpful in accurately identifying the position of an abnormality.

1 *Oblique fissure.* In a normal film the oblique fissure appears as a thin line which extends from the body of the 4th thoracic vertebra across the hilum and down to meet the diaphragm at the anterior 3rd (fig. 6b). With collapse of the lower lobe the oblique fissure is drawn downwards and posteriorly, but with upper lobe collapse the fissure balloons upwards.

2 *Horizontal fissure.* This fissure lies horizontally at the level of the centre of the right hilum and may curve slightly downwards at the anterior end.

3 *Hemidiaphragms.* The left hemidiaphragm is distinguished by the presence of the stomach gas bubble.

4 *Retrosternal air space.* The relatively transradiant area behind the sternum and in front of the heart shadow is often enlarged in severe emphysema as a result of hyperinflation of the lungs.

COMMON ABNORMALITIES

Atelactasis or collapse

Collapse of a lobe is usually evident from the shift of landmarks such as the fissures, mediastinum and blood vessels. Characteristic shadows may be cast by the collapsed lobe itself (fig. 7). Solid structures, such as the heart and diaphragm, which rest against aerated lung, normally appear to have a well-defined margin. When a lobe collapses and the air within is absorbed the clear margin of the adjacent structure disappears. If an upper lobe is collapsed the position of the trachea and mediastinal shadow may shift slightly towards the side of the collapse. If the lower lobe is collapsed there may be slight elevation and loss of definition of the diaphragm and displacement of the heart to that side. The hilar shadow appears smaller on the side of a lobar collapse and as the lobe adjacent to the collapsed lobe occupies more space than normal the vessel markings are more spread out.

The middle lobe lies up against the right heart shadow. On the postero-anterior film the right heart border disappears with collapse of the middle lobe and on a right lateral film it appears as a triangular shadow between the horizontal and oblique fissures. Similarly, the left heart border is lost when the lingula is collapsed. Left lower lobe collapse is characterized by a triangular shadow superimposed on the heart shadow with a well-defined straight line at the lateral margin. With right lower lobe collapse a similar triangular shadow may be superimposed on the right heart, or the shrunken lobe may lie behind the heart shadow. The horizontal fissure is pulled downwards.

Complete collapse of a lung occurs if there is total occlusion of the main bronchus. The lung appears opaque and shrunken as the air within becomes absorbed and the trachea and mediastinum shift *towards* the affected side (fig. 8a).

Consolidation

A consolidated lobe is one in which the alveolar air has been replaced by fluid, cells or cellular exudate and it has an opaque appearance on a radiograph. The dimensions of the lobe remain approxi-

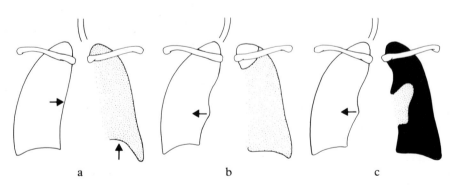

Fig. 8. *Diagrammatic representation of abnormalities seen on radiographs. (a) Total left lung collapse. (b) Large left pleural effusion. (c) Large left pneumothorax. Arrows show direction of mediastinal shift and the change of position of the diaphragm.*

10

mately normal. Patent bronchi may be visible as an air bronchogram.

Pleural effusions

A small pleural effusion may cause blunting of the costophrenic angle. A large effusion casts an opaque shadow with a curved upper edge rising towards the axilla. A very large effusion can obliterate one side of the chest and may produce mediastinal shift *away* from the affected side (fig. 8b).

If fluid is suspected in the pleural space, but is not grossly evident on the ordinary film, it may become apparent if a film is taken with the patient lying on the suspected side (lateral decubitus film). Free fluid moves to the most dependent position. In the supine position the fluid in the most dependent part is lying posteriorly and therefore appears as a generalized haziness over the whole of one lung. In the erect position the fluid will shift to lie in the costophrenic angle and a clear view of the lung will be obtained.

Occasionally fluid is visible in the horizontal fissure on a PA or AP film, but a lateral film is often required to recognize effusions localized within the fissures.

Pleural fluid appears only with a horizontal upper border when air is also present in the pleural space.

Pneumothorax

A large pneumothorax can be identified easily as a clear zone with no vascular markings and a shrunken underlying lung. There will be mediastinal shift *away* from the affected side (fig. 8c). When a pneumothorax is small a fine line shadow marks the edge of the lung and may be difficult to see. A radiograph taken at full expiration makes identification easier by increasing the relative size of the pneumothorax and decreasing the air content (blackness) of the lung.

Bullae

A bulla is a transradiant area containing no vessel markings and with a fine white line of demarcation. Very large bullae cause compression of the unaffected lung tissue with crowding of vascular markings.

Lung abscess

A lung abscess appears as a rounded shadow and may have a fluid level. A lateral film may be necessary to determine the exact position of the abscess.

SPECIAL RADIOGRAPHIC INVESTIGATIONS

Tomography

This is a special radiographic technique in which a series of radiographs can be obtained at different planes through the lung. It is useful in defining tumours and cavities by blurring of the overlying structures such as ribs.

Computerized tomography

Computerized tomography (CT scanning) is another method of producing images of cross sections through any part of the body. The pictures look like slices through the body viewed from the feet of the patient looking towards his head.

CT can distinguish between soft tissues of slightly differing densities and in areas where fat is contained, for example the superior mediastinum, it is useful in detecting lymph nodes. Conventional radiography and tomography often poorly demonstrate pleural disease, subpleural metastases and lesions behind the heart. These may be outlined clearly on a CT scan.

CT is not yet a satisfactory alternative to bronchography in the diagnosis of bronchiectasis, but may be useful where bronchography is contra-indicated (Cooke *et al.* 1987).

Fluoroscopy

Screening, or fluoroscopy is a method of observing movement of the diaphragm during the respiratory cycle. If paralysis of one side of the diaphragm is suspected, the 'sniff' test is carried out. When the patient sniffs the paralysed hemidiaphragm rises, whereas the normal diaphragm moves sharply downwards. This paradoxical upward movement of the paralysed diaphragm is caused by the increased intra-abdominal pressure. Fluoroscopy is also used to identify cardiac abnormalities and shift of the mediastinum by air trapping as may occur if a peanut is inhaled into a bronchus.

Pulmonary angiography

A radio-opaque substance is injected into the bloodstream and radiographs are taken as it passes through the pulmonary circulation, heart and aorta. This is a valuable procedure in the diagnosis of pulmonary embolism alone or in conjunction with radioisotope studies.

Bronchography

A radio-opaque contrast medium is introduced into the trachea, usually under local anaesthesia, either by a nasal catheter or a catheter through the cricothyroid membrane. By varied positioning of the patient the bronchopulmonary segments are lined by the contrast medium. Lateral, oblique and postero-anterior radiographs are taken.

This investigation is used to confirm the diagnosis if bronchiectasis is suspected. The exact site and extent of the bronchial disease can be established (p. 63).

3   Lung sounds

Auscultation is the art of listening to sounds. Listening to and interpreting lung sounds, or the absence of lung sounds, can aid the physiotherapist in the assessment of the patient both before and after treatment.

Coarse changes in lung sounds may be detected by the unaided ear, but a stethoscope will help to localize the source. The stethoscope consists of a diaphragm (for high pitched, high frequency sounds) or bell (for low pitched, low frequency sounds) connected by a length of tubing to two ear pieces. The ear pieces should point slightly forward as they enter the ear and should fit comfortably, but firmly.

Comparative auscultation of areas overlying the bronchopulmonary segments (p. 32) should be made. The patient is asked to breathe deeply, but not noisily through his mouth. This minimizes any sounds which may be produced in his nose.

The classification of lung sounds follows the nomenclature originally stated by Laënnec in the early 19th century when he divided them into the universally accepted normal and bronchial breath sounds. Further divisions have been defined in various ways, but the following can be used as a guideline:

1 *Normal breath sounds* are faint and low pitched. The inspiratory sound is followed, without a pause, by the expiratory sound which soon becomes inaudible and appears comparatively short. Normal sounds, thought to be produced by the turbulent flow of air in the lobar and segmental bronchi (Lehrer 1984), are dampened and lost by the buffering effect of the air filled alveoli.

2 *Bronchial breath sounds* are loud and high pitched. The harsh sounds can be heard throughout inspiration and expiration and there is a pause between the two phases with the expiratory phase being as long or longer than that of inspiration. Areas of consolidation and atelectasis facilitate the transmission of breath sounds to the chest wall. If the bronchi are not patent in an area of consolidation or atelectasis, breath sounds will be absent as there is no direct route for transmission.

3 *Reduced breath sounds* are not necessarily synonomous with reduced ventilation of that part of the lung. Air entry may be normal, that is the bronchi may be patent, but the breath sounds diminished by intervening pathology of the lung or pleura.

4 *Crackles and wheezes* are added, or adventitious sounds.

(a) Crackles (coarse and fine) are discontinuous or explosive sounds often confined to inspiration and thought to be produced by alveoli, bronchioles or bronchi suddenly opening up under an explosive equalization of gas pressure (Forgacs 1978). They may also be attributed to the movement of bronchial secretions in the airways as in bronchitis and bronchiectasis (coarse crackles) and pulmonary oedema. Huffing and coughing may cause disappearance of these sounds or alter their distribution. Crackles are also heard in the absence of excess secretions as in fibrosing alveolitis (fine crackles).

Pleural crackles (pleural rub) are usually localized to a small area and do not disappear or alter with coughing. They are of lower pitch than lung crackles and due to friction between the parietal and visceral pleura, indicating a lesion.

(b) Wheezes are high pitched and low pitched muscial notes produced as air flows through narrowed air passages on the point of collapse analagous to a vibrating reed (Forgacs 1978) and consequently first become apparent during expiration when the airways shorten and narrow. As further narrowing takes place they are also apparent during inspiration.

5 *Stridor* is the crowing noise emanating from the larynx or trachea on inspiration caused by an obstruction in this region.

6 Further information may be gained from *percussion*. This is the firm tapping of the chest wall in order to produce sound vibrations from which the nature of the underlying structures can be detected.

Percussion over a normal chest gives a characteristic resonant note. In pathological conditions the noise may become more or less resonant varying from hyper-resonance to complete dullness. A pneumothorax conveys a hyper-resonant note, but over collapsed or consolidated areas the percussion note is dull and if fluid is present it is 'stony dull'.

4 Breathing control, breathing exercises and postural drainage

BREATHING CONTROL

A common response to breathlessness is to overwork the accessory muscles of respiration with the upper chest and shoulder girdle held in a position of inspiration. Breathing control, or gentle breathing using the lower chest, requires less effort and may relieve breathlessness.

The term diaphragmatic breathing has been used for many years, but lower chest breathing is now known to involve muscle activity in the scalene muscles, the external and internal intercostals, the abdominal muscles and the diaphragm. Breathing control using the lower chest is a more accurate description of this breathing technique. It requires minimal effort in contrast to breathing exercises.

Breathing control:
1 Minimizes the work of breathing.
2 Helps to relieve breathlessness at rest and on exertion.
3 Encourages return to the normal pattern of breathing.
4 Improves ventilation of the bases of the lungs.

To teach breathing control the patient should be positioned so that his back and head are fully supported and his abdominal wall relaxed. If he is in bed, he should sit as high as possible with his knees slightly bent, or if he is out of bed a high-backed chair without arms is most suitable. The physiotherapist's hands rest lightly on the anterior costal margins to stimulate and palpate the movement occurring. Later the patient is instructed to feel the movement himself (fig. 9), but when he has learnt the technique he can relax his hands in a comfortable position.

He breathes out as quietly as possible, while relaxing the shoulders and chest and sinking the lower ribs down and in towards the midline. He is then told to breathe in gently and to 'feel the air coming in round his waist'. The upper

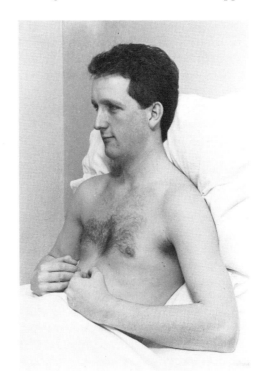

Fig. 9. *Learning breathing control.*

15

chest and shoulders remain relaxed throughout. The emphasis is on gentle breathing with the minimum of effort. The patient should breathe at his own rate and no attempt should be made to slow this down until controlled breathing with the lower chest is achieved. Breathing through the nose is preferable as this warms, moistens and filters the air, but when breathless it is often easier to breathe in and out through the mouth.

A patient who has difficulty learning the pattern of breathing in the sitting position may find it easier to achieve in the high side-lying position (p. 48). It appears that diaphragmatic movement is facilitated in this position as the abdominal viscera cause arching of the dependent portion of the diaphragm and give it a greater potential excursion (Dean 1985).

The patient is closely observed during the training period so that the following common faults may be avoided:

1 *Forced expiration*. With breathing control expiration must be passive. It is important to remember that any forcing or prolongation of expiration will tend to increase airflow obstruction (Donaldson & Gandevia 1962, Gandevia 1963) and increase the work of breathing. In normal expiration the airways shorten and become narrower. If the airways are already partially obstructed and the patient forces expiration, the flow of air will be further impeded. Forced expiration produces a rise in intrapleural pressure and air trapping may result if damaged collapsible airways are compressed by a rise in intrapleural pressure. Forced expiration (huffing) is of value in assisting the removal of secretions in both medical and surgical patients (p. 21), but should be avoided during periods of breathing control.

2 *Prolonged expiration*. Patients should not be encouraged to attempt to empty their lungs to residual volume. The pattern of breathing which follows will be irregular and inefficient and will tend to revert to uncontrolled upper chest breathing with the accessory muscles of respiration overworking.

3 *Trick movements of the abdomen*. The abdominal musculature may be contracted and relaxed without any resultant effect on ventilation.

4 *Over use of the upper chest* and accessory muscles is discouraged, as this will increase the oxygen consumption due to the extra muscle work incurred.

According to the condition of the patient, instruction in breathing control is given in a variety of resting positions as well as while walking up stairs and slopes (p. 47). It is also used as an integral part of a postural drainage treatment.

BREATHING EXERCISES

In contrast to breathing control where the effort of breathing should be minimal, breathing exercises require active work on the part of the patient either during the inspiratory phase or during the expiratory phase according to the particular need. The overall purpose of breathing exercises is to obtain the best possible lung function.

Breathing exercises:
1 Assist in loosening excess bronchial secretions.
2 Assist with removal of the secretions.
3 Aid re-expansion of lung tissue.
4 Mobilize the thoracic cage.
5 Improve ventilation—perfusion relationships.

16

6 May train the respiratory muscles (p. 53 & p. 78).

THORACIC EXPANSION EXERCISES

An increase in lung volume promotes an increase in airflow through the collateral ventilatory channels (p. 4) enabling air to get behind bronchial secretions and assist in loosening them (Menkes & Britt 1980).

Another important concept in explaining the need for breathing exercises emphasizing inspiration is that of 'interdependence' (p. 5). By increasing lung volume, expansion of alveoli is produced. Alveoli exert expanding forces on any collapsed alveoli adjacent to them. Interdependence facilitates homogeneous ventilation and it has been shown that breathing exercises with a 3-second hold at full inspiration are a more efficient method of decreasing atelectasis than breaths without a 'hold' (Ward et al. 1966). This is a useful technique particularly with post-operative patients.

Inspiratory exercises can help to improve movement of the thoracic cage where it is limited by pain or underlying pathology. The term thoracic expansion exercise is used to emphasize movement in a particular area of the rib cage rather than the underlying lung. Changes in ventilation of specific areas of lung by localized exercises is uncertain. In some studies of normal and diseased lungs, localized thoracic exercises have not shown related changes in distribution of ventilation (Grimby et al. 1975, Martin et al. 1976). However, in other studies of normal subjects, the use of various muscle groups for inspiratory exercise have produced an alteration in the distribution of ventilation (Roussos et al. 1977, Fixley et al. 1978).

During both thoracic expansion exercises and breathing control there is activity in the inspiratory muscles of respiration including the diaphragm. The use of the term diaphragmatic breathing instead of breathing control is inaccurate and misleading.

Technique

Pressure is applied to appropriate areas of the chest wall. Utilizing proprioceptive stimuli more effective movement of these areas is obtained. An active inspiration is followed by a relaxed expiration. The patient may be in a half-lying position with the knees slightly flexed over a pillow, or where possible sitting on an upright chair or stool. The physiotherapist should position herself so that she can compare the movement of the two sides of the chest. Alternatively, while lying in an appropriate postural drainage position the patient carries out this breathing exercise to assist in mobilizing secretions (p. 23). There should be a pause for relaxation and breathing control after about four deep breaths or the patient may become dizzy owing to hyperventilation.

Unilaterial lower thoracic expansion

Unilateral lower thoracic expansion is thought to make use of the 'bucket-handle' movement of the ribs.

The physiotherapist places the palm of her hand well round to the side in the mid-axillary line over the 7th, 8th and 9th ribs. The patient should be instructed to relax and to breathe out and to feel the lower ribs sinking down and in. This movement should not be forced. At the end of expiration, the physiotherapist should apply firm pressure to the area described. The patient should be instructed, with the next inspiration to expand the lower ribs against her hand. The pressure should not be excessive, as this could restrict rather than assist the movement. At full inspiration the pressure is released and not reapplied until just before the patient is ready to breathe in again.

When the patient understands the localized movement required, he is taught to apply the pressure himself. This can be done in one of the following ways:

1 With the palm of the hand placed well back in the mid-axillary line (fig. 10). If wrist extension is limited this method is unsuitable.

2 With the back of the fingers. The wrist being held in the mid-position or slight flexion.

3 With the palm of the opposite hand (fig. 11).

Any simulation of costal expansion by side-flexion of the spine should be recognized and corrected and the patient should not be allowed to elevate his shoulder girdle when positioning his hands.

Many patients with obstructive airways disease must first achieve quiet expiration with relaxation of the over-inflated thoracic cage before they attempt basal expansion. The emphasis in surgical patients

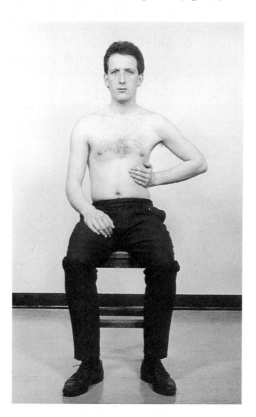

Fig. 10. *Unilateral lower thoracic expansion.*

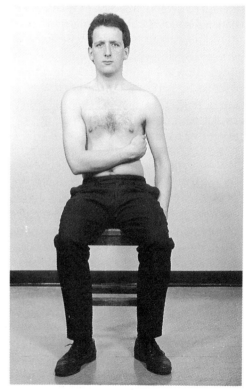

Fig. 11. *Unilateral lower thoracic expansion.*

should be on holding the maximum inspiration for 2–3 seconds before relaxing and breathing out quietly as these patients are known to have a reduced functional residual capacity (p. 80).

Bilateral lower thoracic expansion

Bilateral lower thoracic expansion exercises may be a useful progression of treatment for post-operative patients.

Pressure is applied in the mid-axillary line to both sides of the lower chest with the palms or backs of the hands. The technique used is the same as for unilateral expansion.

It is not advisable to use this exercise for the 'upper chest breather', particularly if the patient is applying his own pressure, as it is difficult to relax the shoulder girdle adequately.

Apical thoracic expansion (fig. 12)

This is useful when there is restricted upper chest movement, for example following gross pleural effusion (p. 74) or incomplete expansion of lung tissue, particularly where there is an apical pneumothorax, for example following lobectomy.

Pressure is applied below the clavicle using the tips of the fingers. The patient breathes in, expanding the chest forwards and upwards against the pressure of the fingers. The shoulders should be relaxed and the expansion held for 2–3 seconds before expiration. If the patient finds this exercise difficult he is instructed to hold his breath for a moment on full inspiration and then to sniff two or three times before breathing out.

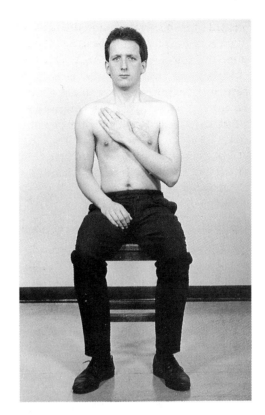

Fig. 12. *Apical thoracic expansion.*

Posterior lower thoracic expansion

When movement is restricted in this area this exercise can be useful.

The patient should sit leaning forward from the hips with a straight back. Pressure is given unilaterally over the posterior aspect of the lower ribs and he can be taught to give this pressure himself.

BELT EXERCISES FOR THORACIC EXPANSION

It may be helpful for the patient to apply his own resistance using a belt. By this method it is possible to relax the shoulder girdle more effectively and many patients practise more conscientiously when a piece of equipment is involved.

Upholstery webbing makes suitable belts for this purpose. The width should be 5–7 cm (2–2.5 in) and the length about 2 metres (6 feet) according to the patient's size.

The patient should be seated on a stool or upright chair and it is often helpful to use a mirror.

Unilateral lower thoracic expansion (fig. 13)

For the left side the belt is placed round the lower chest at the level of the xiphisternum, with a short piece round the left side and held in front with the right hand. The right forearm should be pronated and the wrist in the midline so that the arm is in a relaxed position. The other end is crossed over the thighs and fixed under the left thigh. At the end of the breath out the patient pulls the belt firmly. He then breathes in and expands the left side of the chest outwards against the resistance of the belt. At full inspiration the pressure is released and expansion is maintained for a moment before expiration.

The procedure is reversed for the right side.

Posterior lower thoracic expansion (fig. 14)

The patient should sit leaning forward from the hips with a straight back. For the left side the belt is placed round the back of the chest at the level of the xiphisternum. The piece of belt coming round from the left side is held forwards with the

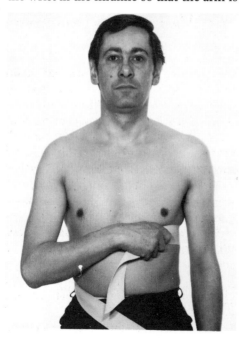

Fig. 13. *Unilateral lower thoracic expansion with belt.*

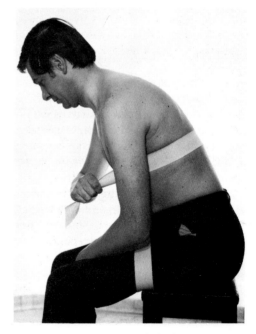

Fig. 14. *Posterior lower thoracic expansion with belt.*

right hand in order to give pressure to the posterior part of the ribs. The other end of the belt is crossed over the thighs and is fixed under the left thigh. At the end of the breath out the patient pulls the belt firmly forwards and he then breathes in and expands the ribs backwards against the resistance of the belt. At full inspiration the pressure is released and expansion is maintained for 2–3 seconds before expiration.

The procedure is reversed for the right side.

THE FORCED EXPIRATION TECHNIQUE

The forced expiration technique is a means of assisting the removal of excess bronchial secretions from the airways. It increases the efficiency of clearance of secretions without causing or increasing bronchospasm (Pryor *et al.* 1979, Pryor & Webber 1979). The technique may be used in a postural drainage position or in any other appropriate position.

The forced expiration technique consists of one or two forced expirations, or huffs, from mid lung volume, followed by a period of relaxation and breathing control (p. 15). When the secretions reach the large airways they are cleared by a huff or cough at a high lung volume. The periods of breathing control (fig. 15), after huffs or coughs, are essential to prevent the possible occurrence of bronchospasm or to avoid increase in bronchospasm if it is already present.

A forced expiratory manoeuvre produces compression and narrowing within the airways from a point dependent on lung volume (the equal pressure point) (Mead *et al.* 1967). At high lung volume

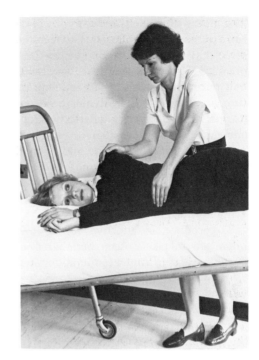

Fig. 15. *Breathing control. By courtesy of Physiotherapy.*

this point lies in the trachea and main bronchi. Under normal circumstances bronchial secretions are effectively cleared from this region by coughing or huffing at a high lung volume. As the lung volume decreases the point at which this dynamic compression takes place moves further down the bronchial tree (Leith 1968) and is accompanied by a rapid vibratory movement of the bronchial wall. Progressively deeper portions of the airways can therefore be cleared. In the absence of chest disease the narrowing is evenly distributed, but in patients with airways obstruction it may be more marked and unevenly distributed.

To produce a cough, a forced expiratory effort is made against a closed glottis causing a rise in intrathoracic pressure.

21

The glottis then opens abruptly so that a large pressure gradient exists between the alveolar pressure and the upper tracheal pressure (now atmospheric). A very rapid flow results. The high intrathoracic pressure inverts the posterior membrane of the intrathoracic trachea and narrows it to one-sixth of its normal area (Comroe 1965) (figs. 16 & 17). The rapid flow, combined with this narrowing, increases the explosive force of the air which dislodges mucus and foreign particles bringing them to the pharynx.

To produce an effective cough it is important to take a deep breath before coughing and to contract the abdominal

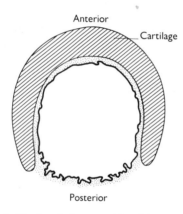

Fig. 16. *Trachea during normal breathing.*

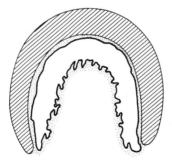

Fig. 17. *Trachea during cough—internal area reduced to one-sixth of its normal area.*

muscles during the cough. After two or three coughs a period of breathing control should follow, or if another deep breath is taken, the patient should not be allowed to go into an uncontrolled paroxysm of coughing as this is exhausting. If the patient persists in coughing without breathing in, cough syncope may occur. Relaxation and breathing control should be interspersed between short bouts of coughing.

To produce a huff a forced expiratory effort is made, but the glottis remains open and the intrathoracic pressure does not rise to such high levels. The intrathoracic pressure generated again compresses and narrows the intrathoracic trachea and bronchi and an increased expiratory flow is achieved. Mucus and foreign particles are dislodged and moved up the bronchial tree.

It has been shown that the mean maximum transpulmonary pressure during voluntary coughing is greater than during forced expiration (Langlands 1967). A cough in patients with airflow obstruction therefore produces greater compression and narrowing of the airways than a huff. This sudden airway collapse limits flow and reduces the efficiency of the cough in bronchial clearance. This, combined with clinical observations that a series of coughs without intervening inspirations is more exhausting than a single continuous huff down to the same lung volume, is further evidence to support the use of the huff.

In attempting to clear secretions from the smaller airways, a huff started at mid lung volume and continued down to low lung volume is the most efficient. After taking a medium sized breath in, the patient breathes out forcefully through the mouth, contracting the abdominal muscles at the same time. Instructing the patient to *'squeeze the air out'* is often helpful. Breathing out loudly with a partially closed larynx or just clearing the back of the throat does not produce an effective huff. Children as young as 3 years old can be taught to huff, but may need to practise by blowing through a tube (Thompson 1978) (fig. 18). Adults having difficulty in producing a correct huff also find a tube, such as a disposable peak expiratory flow mouthpiece, helpful. If a patient complains of a sore throat, the technique is being carried out incorrectly.

The huff has to be taught carefully and adapted to suit the individual patient. It must be long enough to move the more peripheral secretions, but not so long or so forceful that it becomes a paroxysm of coughing. When copious proximal secretions are present a huff will promote coughing immediately, but having cleared these secretions the aim of the forced expiration technique is to move the more peripheral secretions gradually without incessant and tiring bouts of coughing. It is not essential to start the huff at mid lung volume, but it is a waste of energy to take a full breath in when it is only the part of the huff to a low lung volume that is having the effect of moving the more peripheral secretions. A child may find it easier to learn the technique by taking a deep breath in before huffing the air out.

POSTURAL DRAINAGE

The patient is positioned to allow gravity to assist the drainage of secretions from specific areas of the lungs. The positions are based on the anatomy of the bronchial tree as shown in the diagrams (fig. 29, p. 32). The value of postural drainage, in

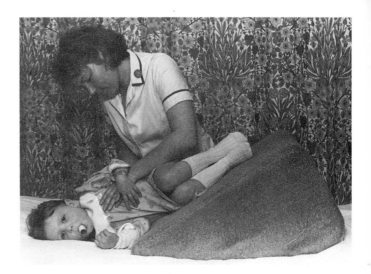

Fig. 18. *Learning to huff through a tube in the mouth.*

the clearance of excess bronchial secretions, has been established (Cochrane *et al.* 1977, Bateman *et al.* 1979) and using the techniques described below an improvement in lung function has been shown (Webber *et al.* 1986). The importance of using gravity assisted positions, in patients with excess bronchial secretions, has been demonstrated (Sutton *et al.* 1983, Hofmeyr *et al.* 1986).

Appropriate positioning should be accompanied by active participation and requires the patient's full concentration. The treatment is ineffective if the patient lies passively in a postural drainage position except in the rare circumstances of pooling of bronchial secretions in lung abscess or in occasional cases of bronchiectasis.

Breathing techniques available to assist clearance of bronchial secretions are:
1 *Thoracic expansion exercises.* These exercises assist in loosening bronchial secretions (p. 17).
2 *Breathing control.* This prevents hyperventilation and fatigue.

23

3 *The forced expiration technique.* The huffs assist clearance of secretions and the periods of relaxation and breathing control and prevent the possibility of an increase in airflow obstruction (p. 21).

These techniques are used as a cycle, in any appropriate position and may be accompanied by chest percussion and/or vibratory chest shaking.

PERCUSSION

Percussion of the chest wall produces an energy wave which is transmitted through the chest wall to the airways. This mechanical effect may loosen mucus from the bronchial walls and appears to be more effective when combined with thoracic expansion exercises than with breathing at tidal volume. Chest percussion is most often the manual technique of clapping, but mechanical devices are sometimes employed.

Clapping is carried out with the hands slightly cupped and by quick, relaxed flexion and extension of the wrists (Fig. 19). It should be performed over clothes or a towel as it is not intended to stimulate the skin and it should never be painful.

There is no doubt that gentle clapping is necessary to stimulate coughing in infants and children, as treatment has to be passive until the child is old enough to actively use the breathing techniques, huffing and coughing. This can be performed using the finger tips of one hand in small infants, or by application to the chest wall of a small cushioned face mask fitted onto the index or middle finger (see fig. 108, p. 150). The latter has been shown to be a comfortable and effective method of chest percussion in infants (Tudehope & Bagley 1980, p. 149).

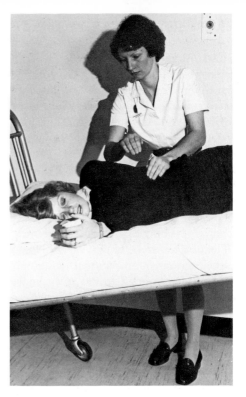

Fig. 19. *Clapping.*

A reduction in forced expiratory volume in 1 second (FEV_1) following chest percussion has been reported (Campbell *et al.* 1975 & Wollmer *et al.* 1985), but this has not occurred when pauses for relaxation and breathing control have been interspersed during the postural drainage treatment (Pryor & Webber 1979). Patients with severe bronchospasm do not benefit from physiotherapy to assist removal of secretions until some bronchodilation has taken place. When bronchospasm is less severe, clapping may be helpful and it is found that a slow rate of clapping (approximately 60 beats/minute) which can be performed with one hand, is more relaxing than a faster speed.

In some countries percussion is not used in the belief that it causes a fall in arterial oxygen tension. A study on acute patients in an intensive care unit showed this effect (Connors *et al.* 1980), but studies on chronic respiratory patients have shown no fall in oxygen tension with chest percussion (May & Munt 1979). Provided that treatment is accompanied by breathing exercises, relaxation and breathing control, percussion appears to do no harm. Its benefits have yet to be proved.

Many patients are able to do self-clapping (fig. 20). This is more effective using one hand than both hands because it avoids elevation of the shoulder girdle on the side of the uppermost arm and allows the patient to concentrate more easily on the accompanying breathing exercises.

In stable chronic respiratory patients it has been shown that self-clapping does not increase sputum production beyond that obtained by the inspiratory breathing exercises alone (fig. 21) (Webber *et al.* 1985). It should therefore not be considered an essential part of a self-postural drainage treatment. Some patients who have been using clapping for many years feel that it is beneficial and will prefer to continue to use it.

There are several *mechanical percussors* available, but there is no evidence at present to suggest that bronchial secretions are cleared more efficiently when using one of these devices.

In the adolescent and adult patient with cystic fibrosis, carrying out his own treatment, it has been shown that a mechanical percussor gives no additional benefit if postural drainage is combined with the forced expiration technique (Pryor *et al.* 1981).

The high frequency oscillator is another

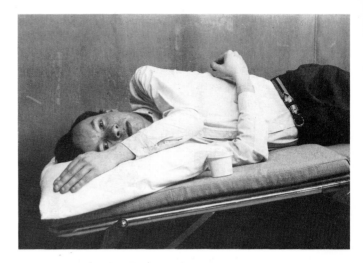

Fig. 20. *Self-clapping combined with lower thoracic expansion exercises. By courtesy of the Cystic Fibrosis Research Trust.*

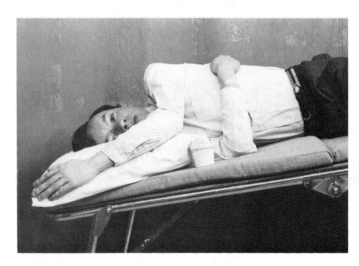

Fig. 21. *Lower thoracic expansion during postural drainage.*

mechanical device which may assist in clearance of secretions. Oral high frequency oscillations are superimposed on normal tidal breathing (George *et al.* 1985a & 1985b). It is not yet known whether this device offers any advantage

25

over the breathing techniques used with postural drainage and it is under investigation. It is possible that it may relieve breathlessness in the severely disabled respiratory patient.

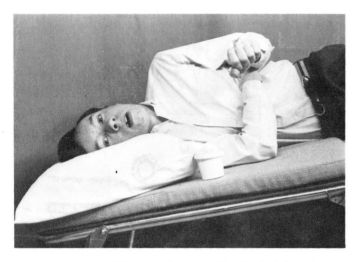

Fig. 22. *Self-compression with a huff. By courtesy of the Cystic Fibrosis Research Trust.*

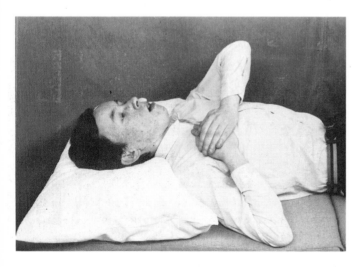

Fig. 23. *Self-compression of the anterior segment of the right upper lobe.*

VIBRATORY CHEST SHAKING

Mechanical energy is again transmitted through the chest wall. The manoeuvre is performed only during the expiratory phase of breathing and therefore has the added effect of increasing the expiratory flow rate.

Relaxed hands are placed on the appropriate area of the thorax and by using her body weight the physiotherapist produces a vibratory shaking of the chest wall during expiration. Shaking is combined with the relaxed expiration of the thoracic expansion exercises and can also be used to reinforce the effect of the forced expiration technique in clearing excess bronchial secretions. Many patients are able to assist their own postural drainage by giving compression over the lateral aspect of the chest wall using the hand of the underneath arm and the upper arm and elbow of the uppermost arm (fig. 22). Self-compression, over the midzones or the anterior segments of the upper lobes, can be used when draining these areas (fig. 23). On completion of a period of postural drainage, self-compression can be useful in the sitting position. The arms are folded across the chest and pressure is applied in conjunction with a huff (fig. 24). Not all patients find benefit from self-compression, but having perfected the forced expiration technique, instruction in self-compression may be given and the patient can decide if it gives additional help.

Treatment programme for postural drainage

The aim of a postural drainage treatment is to clear secretions as effectively as possible without the patient suffering

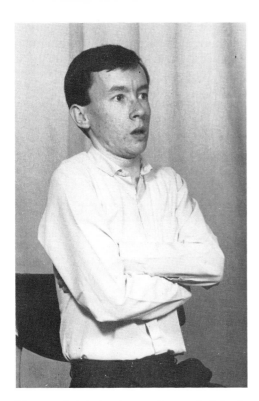

Fig. 24. *Completing the treatment—a huff in the sitting position.*

lung are affected, it may not be possible to drain all of them in one session. Different areas can be drained at different times.

Many patients like to have a programme outlined for the postural drainage session. While the physiotherapist is with the patient she will give assistance, but if she leaves the patient at intervals he should continue the active treatment. The programme must be adapted to each individual's requirements, but an example is:
(a) Three or four thoracic expansion exercises which may be combined with clapping or shaking (by an assistant or the patient himself).
(b) Pause for relaxation and breathing control (fig. 25).
(c) The forced expiration technique: one or two huffs followed by a pause for breathing control.

When secretions reach the upper airways another huff or cough is added, followed by breathing control, before returning to the thoracic expansion exercises. This cycle is repeated until the area being drained is clear.

discomfort or becoming exhausted. All patients who are able to cooperate should carry out cycles of the breathing techniques which can be accompanied by chest percussion, vibratory shaking or compression, if they are found to be helpful, performed either by the physiotherapist or the patient himself.

Each appropriate postural drainage position should ideally be maintained until the affected area is clear of secretions. The length of time required varies with each individual, but with active treatment an area is usually cleared in 10–20 minutes. Postural drainage may be required 1–5 times a day according to the patient's condition. If several areas of the

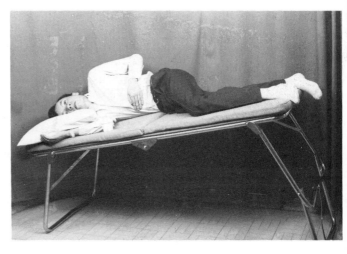

Fig. 25. *Breathing control during self postural drainage. By courtesy of the Cystic Fibrosis Research Trust.*

27

It is useful, with many patients, to give an objective point at which treatment may be stopped. A minimum of 10 minutes for a productive area should be carried out and when the patient cannot detect any secretions with a huff of correct length, during two consecutive cycles of the breathing techniques, the position can be changed.

It must be emphasized that rushing treatment, by shortening or omitting the pauses for breathing control, will make treatment ineffective. The airways constrict with forced expiratory manoeuvres and it is essential to relax and allow the airways to open again.

To complete the treatment the patient can sit on the edge of the bed, or on a chair and clear any remaining secretions from the upper airways by using the huff with or without chest compression (fig. 24).

It is inadvisable to carry out postural drainage immediately after a meal as the patient may tend to feel nauseous or even vomit and will not perform the treatment adequately. Postural drainage is also unsuitable immediately before a meal because the patient may feel too tired to enjoy his food. Some patients find it easier to cough productively after having a drink.

Postural drainage at home

Many patients who require postural drainage at home are able to carry out their treatment independently and efficiently using the cycle of breathing techniques. Others who are more disabled will benefit from clapping and chest shaking given by an assistant in conjunction with the breathing techniques. When teaching relatives or friends how to clap and shake the chest, it is essential that they understand the necessity for the periods of relaxation and breathing control.

Patients who are too frail to manage chest compression and have no one to assist at home, are able to move secretions by effective huffs. The vibratory action of the posterior membrane of the trachea and main bronchi, in addition to the dynamic compression of the airways during the forced expiratory manoeuvre, promote movement of the secretions. The postural drainage positions, where the patient is lying prone, make self-clapping and chest compression difficult, but independent treatment can be successful by means of the cycle of breathing techniques.

A patient who is in hospital and who needs to continue postural drainage at home, often benefits from carrying out his own treatment for 1 or 2 days prior to discharge. The physiotherapist, having carefully instructed the patient, supervises the treatment during these last days and by this means he gains the confidence required to know that he can manage without help at home. The areas requiring drainage and the time needed for treatment must be discussed with each patient. In most cases treatment will be required for at least 15–20 minutes, twice daily.

The means of positioning the patient at home must be established. It is difficult for the majority of patients to elevate the foot of the bed at home. Some patients have a bed in a spare room that they keep in a tipped position. Others have a frame to tilt the whole body to a suitable angle (fig. 26a). A simple, but less comfortable method is to lie over firm cushions arranged in the centre of the bed or on the floor (fig. 26b). The patient can lie over these in varying positions to drain several areas of the lungs. Alternatively, a firm wedge of polyether foam can be obtained, but this is only suitable for children and light adults.

Motivating patients to carry out treatment regularly on a long-term basis is not easy. It is therefore important to organize a means of drainage that is comfortable, effective and does not require preparation time. It may be necessary to arrange for the loan of a frame at home. Although for simplicity some of the frames tip only to an angle of 15°, this is found to be adequate for draining both the mid and lower zones if the frame is firm. However, if an extra depth of tip is required, a pillow can be placed under the pelvis. The deep tipping position that has been used with the patients lying over the side of the bed is unsuitable. Most patients find it uncomfortable and it drains more specifically the posterior basal segments of the lower lobes.

Small children and infants can be given postural drainage by placing them over the knee (fig. 27). It is usually preferable to give this treatment immediately prior to a feed.

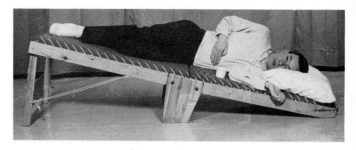

Fig. 26a. *Frame for postural drainage at home.*

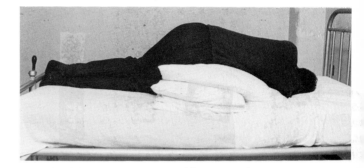

Fig. 26b. *Pillows used for postural drainage at home.*

Modified postural drainage

Some patients suffer from orthopnoea and cannot lie flat without becoming dyspnoeic. If a patient has excess secretions at the lung bases and is likely to become distressed by orthodox postural drainage positions, it is better to compromise and to position him in a high side-lying position or as flat as possible, on alternate sides, without tipping the foot of the bed. In this position the cycle of breathing techniques, combined with clapping and shaking can be given as usual. If this position does not cause distress, the foot of the bed can be elevated slightly at the next treatment.

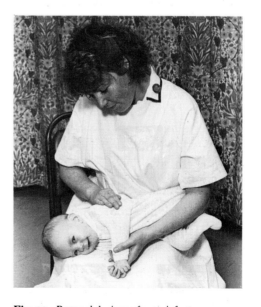

Fig. 27. *Postural drainage for an infant.*

Adjuncts to postural drainage

Bronchodilators. If a bronchodilator has been prescribed, this should be used before postural drainage.

Humidification. When secretions are tenacious, or airways plugged, additional high humidity is helpful preceding postural drainage. This can be administered by means of a humidifier or nebulizer containing sterile water or normal saline (p. 138). Heated humidification should be used in patients with reversible airflow obstruction.

Mucolytic agents. If prescribed, mucolytic agents should be used before postural drainage. They are of uncertain benefit and should be used with caution. Some mucolytics have an irritant effect producing hypersecretion and may cause bronchospasm.

IPPB. Patients with tenacious secretions and poor chest movement who have not responded to the treatments described, or those who become exhausted even during short treatments, may benefit by using IPPB in conjunction with postural drainage (p. 120).

PEP. The device to give positive expiratory pressure (PEP) consists of a mask and a one-way valve system to which an appropriate resistance is applied in the expiratory limb. PEP is sometimes used instead of thoracic expansion exercises as it is thought to mobilize bronchial secretions. Patients who were relying on a relative at home to assist with postural drainage, found it more effective to do their treatment without an assistant using PEP in the sitting position (Falk *et al.* 1984), but patients treating themselves by using the active cycle of breathing techniques in postural drainage positions have found no advantage in the use of PEP (Hofmeyr *et al.* 1986).

Contra-indications to postural drainage, clapping and shaking

Contra-indications to postural drainage include the following conditions: recent severe haemoptysis, severe hypertension, cerebral oedema, aortic and cerebral aneurysms, cardiovascular instability where arrhythmias or pulmonary oedema are present and conditions of the oesophagus or diaphragm causing gastric reflux. In many cases of acute asthma and severe emphysema, dyspnoea would be increased by postural drainage for the lung bases and a modified position is used.

Neither clapping nor chest shaking are painful procedures if they are carried out skilfully. The pressure exerted on the thorax must be modified according to the build of the patient as well as the chest condition. A patient with osteoporosis or metastatic deposits affecting the ribs or vertebral column must be treated gently.

Other contra-indications to clapping, mechanical percussion and shaking include haemoptysis, acute pleuritic pain and active pulmonary tuberculosis. Provided that thoracic expansion exercises, the forced expiration technique and coughing are carried out effectively, clapping and vibrations are rarely indicated for adults following cardio-thoracic surgery. If a patient is mechanically ventilated, vibrations or chest shaking may be required (p. 111).

Recording of sputum

Measurements of sputum weight are helpful in assessing response to treatment and progress of a patient. Twenty-four hour weight of sputum may be recorded on the patient's progress chart by the nursing staff on the ward, but it is useful for the physiotherapist to make objective measurements herself.

The following scheme for the visual grading of sputum may be useful:

M1 = mucoid with no suspicion of pus
M2 = predominantly mucoid with a suspicion of pus
P1 = one-third purulent, two-thirds mucoid
P2 = two-thirds purulent, one-third mucoid
P3 = more than two-thirds purulent (Miller 1963)
FB = fresh blood staining
OB = old blood staining
R = rusty (p. 62).

Bronchography

If there appears to be an excessive quantity of secretions which could prevent adequate outlining of the bronchi by the contrast medium in a bronchogram, the patient should be given appropriate postural drainage before the procedure.

After a bronchogram (fig. 28) the majority of the contrast medium is sucked into the peripheral bronchi during inspiration and is gradually absorbed into the blood stream. The contrast medium remaining in the upper airways is removed by the action of the cilia and effective huffing and coughing. Although postural drainage is not essential for a patient with normal airways a brief session, with assistance from a physiotherapist immediately following the procedure, makes the patient more comfortable.

Postural drainage is required for those patients with bronchiectasis. The contrast medium is unlikely to be sucked as far into the periphery because of the blockage of the small airways by sputum and endobronchial disease. The cilia are usually

destroyed in these bronchiectatic airways and postural drainage speeds up the procedure of clearing the contrast medium from the bronchi.

It is important that patients have nothing to eat or drink for at least 3 hours after a bronchogram, until the effect of the local anaesthetic has worn off.

If the bronchogram has been performed through the cricothyroid membrane, the patient is instructed to give pressure with a finger over the cricothyroid cartilage whenever he huffs or coughs, for at least 6 hours after the procedure, to avoid subcutaneous (surgical) emphysema.

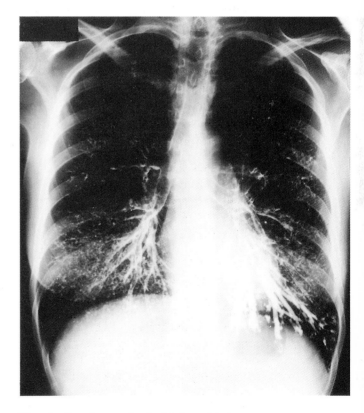

Fig. 28. *Bronchogram showing left lower lobe bronchiectasis.*

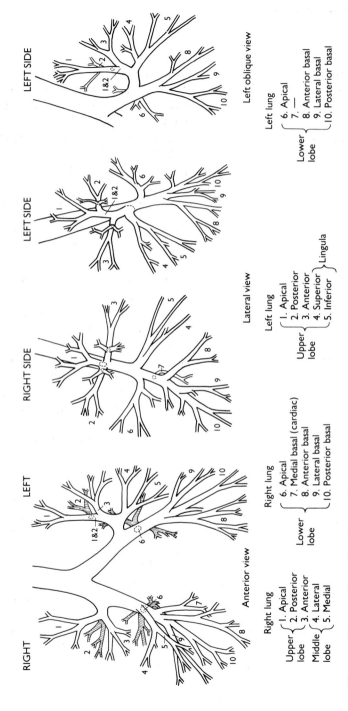

Fig. 29. *Diagram illustrating the bronchopulmonary nomenclature approved by the Thoracic Society. Reproduced by permission of the Editors of Thorax.*

Postural drainage positions

(figs. 30–40)

LOBE		POSTURE
Upper lobe	**1** Apical bronchus	**1** Sitting upright with slight variations according to the position of the lesion, i.e. slightly leaning backwards, forwards or sideways.
	2 Posterior bronchus (a) Right	**2a** Lying on the left side horizontally and then turned 45° on to the face, resting against a pillow, with another supporting the head.
	(b) Left	**b** Lying on the right side turned 45° on to the face, with three pillows arranged to lift the shoulders 30 cm (12 in) from the bed.
	3 Anterior bronchus	**3** Lying supine with the knees slightly flexed.
Lingula	**4** Superior bronchus	**4 & 5** Lying supine with the body a quarter turned to the right maintained by a pillow under the left side from shoulder to hip. Foot of the bed raised 35 cm (14 in): chest tilted to an angle of 15°.
	5 Inferior bronchus	
Middle lobe	**4** Lateral bronchus	**4 & 5** Lying supine with the body a quarter turned to the left maintained by a pillow under the right side from shoulder to hip. Foot of the bed raised 35 cm (14 in): chest tilted to an angle of 15°.
	5 Medial bronchus	
Lower lobe	**6** Apical bronchus	**6** Lying prone with a pillow under the abdomen.
	7 Medial basal (cardiac) bronchus	**7** Lying on the right side with a pillow under the hips. Foot of the bed raised 45 cm (18 in): chest tilted to an angle of 20°.
	8 Anterior basal bronchus	**8** Lying supine with the buttocks resting on a pillow and the knees flexed. Foot of the bed raised 45 cm (18 in): chest tilted to an angle of 20°.
	9 Lateral basal bronchus	**9** Lying on the opposite side with a pillow under the hips. Foot of the bed raised 45 cm (18 in): chested tilted to an angle of 20°.
	10 Posterior basal bronchus	**10** Lying prone with a pillow under the hips. Foot of the bed raised 45 cm (18 in): chest tilted to an angle of 20°.

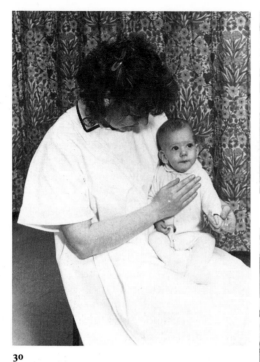

30

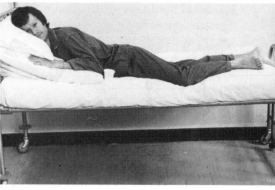

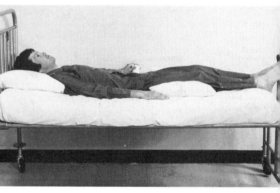

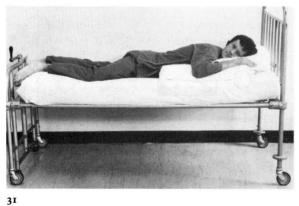

31

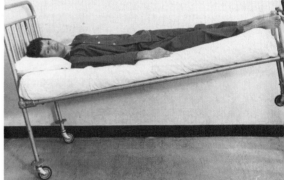

Fig. 30. *Apical segment left upper lobe.*
Fig. 31. *Posterior segment right upper lobe.*

Fig. 32. *Posterior segment left upper lobe.*
Fig. 33. *Anterior segments upper lobes.*
Fig. 34. *Lingula.*

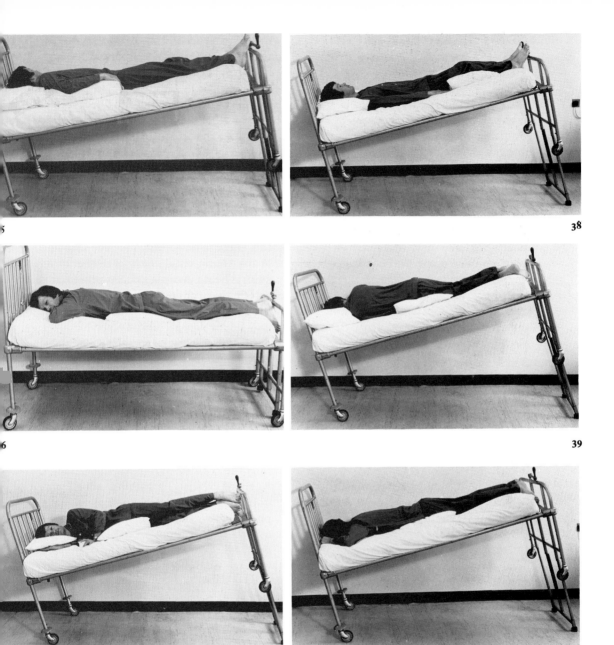

Fig. 35. *Right middle lobe.*
Fig. 36. *Apical segments lower lobes.*
Fig. 37. *Right medial basal and left lateral basal segments lower lobes.*

Fig. 38. *Anterior basal segments lower lobes.*
Fig. 39. *Lateral basal segment right lower lobe.*
Fig. 40. *Posterior basal segments lower lobes.*

POSITIONING FOR IMPROVED VENTILATION AND PERFUSION

Positioning, in gravity assisted positions, is necessary to assist clearance of excess bronchial secretions, but when secretions are not a treatment priority it may be useful to consider positioning a patient to improve oxygenation of the arterial blood.

Gravity has been shown to have an important effect on pulmonary gas exchange in spontaneously breathing adults. Studies have demonstrated that both ventilation and perfusion are preferentially distributed towards the dependent lung during quiet breathing. In sick patients with unilateral lung disease, gas exchange may be improved by positioning such patients in side-lying with the unaffected lung dependent (Zack *et al.* 1974). In bilateral lung disease arterial oxygen tension has been shown to be higher with the patient lying on his right side than on his left side. This is probably due to cardiac compression of the left lung or the smaller volume of the left lung (Zack *et al.* 1974).

With infants and very young children, in the side-lying position, it has been shown that ventilation is preferentially distributed to the upper-most lung. To obtain the best oxygenation with unilateral lung disease the infant should be nursed with the unaffected lung upper-most (Davies *et al.* 1985). Two reasons for this difference between adults and infants have been postulated. Closure of peripheral airways is more likely to occur in infants in the dependent lung because the chest wall is floppy and does not provide as much support to the lungs as in adults. The weight of the abdominal contents in adults in the side-lying position, provides a preferential load on the dependent diaphragm improving its contractility, whereas the smaller size of the abdomen in infants and young children does not have this effect. The age at which the situation of the young child changes to that of an adult is being investigated. At present it is certain that a child of up to 2 years old has the reverse situation of the adult, but it may be for considerably longer.

In adults who are paralysed or those anaesthetized and receiving intermittent positive pressure ventilation, where the advantage of diaphragmatic loading has been removed, the usual increase in ventilation to the dependent lung is also reversed (Rehder *et al.* 1972).

Thus it is important to consider carefully the position of hypoxaemic patients. A spontaneously breathing adult with unilateral lung disease, such as an acute pneumonia, should benefit by being nursed with the unaffected lung dependent, while an infant should be nursed with the unaffected lung uppermost.

5 Oxygen therapy

Oxygen therapy is often required in the management of patients with chest disease, but it is important to control the concentration of oxygen in many clinical circumstances.

An understanding of when oxygen must be prescribed with caution requires some knowledge of the normal chemical control of breathing.

In health, the level of the arterial carbon dioxide tension is the most important single factor controlling the rate and depth of breathing. A variety of mechanisms stimulate breathing when metabolic requirements are increased, as for example during exercise and the level of carbon dioxide in the arterial blood remains surprisingly constant. An increase in this level beyond the normal range causes a sensation of severe breathlessness and stimulates the healthy person to hyperventilate vigorously, so removing the excess carbon dioxide and restoring the level to normal.

Some chronic lung diseases are characterized by the patient's tendency to breathe inadequately, the work of breathing is excessive and the efficiency of gas exchange is lowered by airflow obstruction. An example of such a condition is chronic bronchitis with secondary emphysema. If breathing is inadequate, the level of carbon dioxide in the arterial blood ($Pa\text{co}_2$) tends to rise and the level of oxygen ($Pa\text{o}_2$) tends to fall (normal range, $Pa\text{o}_2$: 9·3–14·0 kPa, 70–105 mm Hg, $Pa\text{co}_2$: 4·8–5·6 kPa, 36–42 mm Hg). The respiratory centre slowly becomes acclimatized to the abnormally high level of carbon dioxide in the arterial blood and no longer responds by stimulating an increase in the rate and depth of breathing. When the respiratory centre no longer matches respiratory effort to the patient's requirements, the only stimulus which keeps the patient breathing regularly is the lack of oxygen (hypoxia) in the blood.

Hypoxia is dangerous because many organs, for example the heart and kidneys, suffer from oxygen lack. If hypoxia is relieved by the administration of high concentrations of oxygen, the last effective stimulus to respiration is removed and breathing becomes progressively more shallow and ineffective, so allowing the carbon dioxide level to rise even further. The elevated carbon dioxide level, hypercapnia, renders the patient drowsy and uncooperative and eventually comatose. He is unable to cough and secretions accumulate in the lungs adding to his respiratory disability. The oxygen lack has been relieved so he retains a 'good' colour and often looks unusually flushed and hot because of the effects of excess carbon dioxide on the skin. This condition is very dangerous and may be fatal.

The administration of *low* concentrations of oxygen (24–35%) will partly relieve the hypoxia, reducing the risk of damage to the vital organs without completely eliminating the stimulus to breathe. The level of carbon dioxide may rise a little when even low concentrations of oxygen are used, but in many patients it is possible to reach an equilibrium position in which both carbon dioxide and oxygen levels in the blood are acceptable. This is best achieved by serial measurement of blood gas values. The patient would be observed for deterioration in conscious level or ability to cough and cooperate. Any deterioration in the mental state indicates that excessive oxygen has been used and the concentration must be adjusted. If a satisfactory position cannot be achieved or if serious hypoxia persists in spite of all attempts to remove secretions and relieve spasm, intubation and intermittent positive pressure ventilation (IPPV) are generally necessary.

Not all patients with chronic lung disease respond in this way. In acute asthma, the patient may breathe even more deeply or frequently than is necessary to maintain the normal level of carbon dioxide in the blood, in an attempt to relieve the hypoxia which is always a common feature of the condition.

In the older age groups, or those with chronic asthma and in all patients when fatigued, this ability to hyperventilate is lost and inadequate ventilation and elevation of the carbon dioxide level in the blood may follow. Until this stage is reached, most patients with asthma benefit from oxygen in high concentrations.

In another group of disorders (pulmonary oedema, fibrosing alveolitis, sarcoidosis and pulmonary embolism) the ability to absorb oxygen is impaired to a much greater degree than the ability to excrete carbon dioxide, largely because a considerable percentage of the pulmonary blood flows to parts of the lung which are not being properly ventilated. The 'good' areas of lung compensate for the 'bad' in terms of carbon dioxide removal, but not for the uptake of oxygen owing to the different diffusing capacities of carbon dioxide and oxygen. These patients are always very breathless. They generally breathe more deeply and frequently than is necessary to maintain a normal carbon dioxide level, in an attempt to relieve the hypoxia. They require high concentrations of oxygen and there is no risk of respiratory depression because the respiratory centre does not lose its normal sensitivity to carbon dioxide.

A variety of masks is available to provide oxygen therapy. The masks which operate on the venturi or jet mixing principle provide a controlled percentage of oxygen (fixed performance devices (Sykes *et al.* 1976)). The high flow exceeds the patient's peak inspiratory flow rate. The entrained room air provides some humidity, but additional humidification can be obtained by an adapter fitted over the air-entraining holes and connected by wide bore tubing to a humidifier (p. 137).

Nasal cannulae and masks which do not utilize the venturi principle (variable performance devices) deliver dry oxygen unless some form of humidification is placed in the circuit. Compressed oxygen bubbled through water obtains some moisture, but much of this is lost by condensation in narrow bore tubing before it reaches the patient. To provide more effective humidification, wide bore tubing must connect the oxygen mask to a humidifier. Wide bore tubing cannot be connected to nasal cannulae, but clinically a bubble humidifier and narrow bore tubing prevents uncomfortable drying of the nasal mucosa.

If a patient is receiving oxygen therapy, the mask should not be removed during breathing exercises or postural drainage except for expectoration. When continuous oxygen therapy has been prescribed, the mask can be replaced by nasal cannulae during meals. For patient comfort, nasal cannulae must be run at low flow rates, usually 2 litres/minute.

Oxygen may be used to drive an intermittent positive pressure breathing (IPPB) apparatus for treatment in conjunction with physiotherapy. With many of these machines, the percentage of oxygen received by the patient will be considerably higher than the controlled percentage delivered by the appropriate venturi mask (fig. 41), for example in the treatment of the chronic bronchitic. This higher percentage is rarely dangerous during treatment, because the patient's ventilation is assisted and the removal of secretions from the chest as a result of treatment often leads to an improvement in the general condition. It has been suggested that a few patients become more drowsy during or after IPPB treatment because of the high percentage of oxygen received. A study has shown that increased drowsiness (caused by hypercapnia) can occur whether oxygen or air is used to power the IPPB device and that this deterioration is not dependent on the driving gas, but on inappropriate setting of the ventilator. The pressure and flow controls must be set to provide an adequate tidal volume, particular attention being required when treating patients with a rigid thoracic cage (Starke et al. 1979).

When treating patients with severe hypoxia, for example acute asthma, fibrosing alveolitis or left ventricular failure, oxygen is required and it is dangerous to use IPPB driven entirely by compressed air. Thus IPPB should be powered either by compressed oxygen with the air entrainment device in use, or by compressed air with an attachment to provide a controlled, optimal concentration of added oxygen.

When inhaling drugs from a nebulizer, without IPPB, the patient is breathing spontaneously. Oxygen to power the nebulizer could be dangerous in the case of a hypercapnic patient and the nebulizer should be powered by air (p. 132).

Long-term domiciliary oxygen therapy has been shown to improve the length and quality of life in selected patients with severe chronic airflow limitation (Nocturnal Oxygen Therapy Trial Group 1980, Medical Research Council Working Party 1981). The expected gradual progression of pulmonary hypertension associated with this condition is arrested, or at least slowed down, by use of long-term oxygen therapy. This benefit will not occur unless

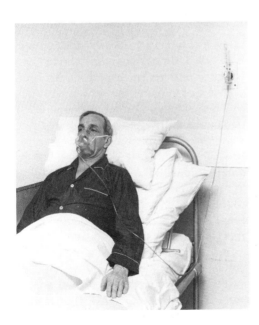

Fig. 41. *Venturi mask for oxygen therapy.*

39

oxygen is used at a low flow for a minimum of 15 hours/day and should be prescribed only for carefully selected patients.

An oxygen concentrator (fig. 42) is a more cost-effective and convenient method for providing domiciliary oxygen than cylinders (Evans *et al.* 1983). Simple plastic tubing should be fitted in areas of the home to allow maximum mobility for the patient.

Portable oxygen (fig. 43) may relieve breathlessness and possibly increase exercise tolerance in some patients (p. 52). Portable cylinders cannot be filled from an oxygen concentrator and must be filled from a larger cylinder. This can be a frightening and difficult procedure and the patient should be given careful instruction and opportunity to practise under supervision.

The most common method of administration of oxygen at home is through nasal

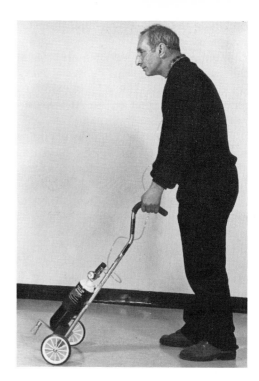

Fig. 43. *Portable oxygen.*

cannulae, but transtracheal oxygen delivery is a practical technique which some patients find more cosmetically acceptable. A micro-catheter is inserted into the trachea so that most of the anatomical deadspace is bypassed and the oxygen requirement, compared to nasal cannulae, is reduced (Banner & Govan 1986). Portable cylinders hold such a limited supply of oxygen that this reduction in flow requirement may be an advantage for some severely disabled patients. However, great care must be taken to avoid infection with the transtracheal method of delivery.

It is important to remember that oxygen is a drug and must, like all drugs, be carefully used so that undesirable side-effects may be avoided.

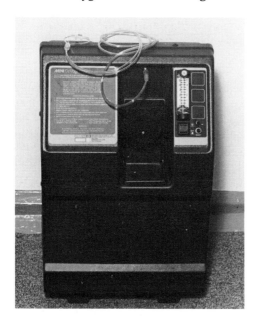

Fig. 42. *An oxygen concentrator.*

6 Medical conditions

TYPES OF DISABILITY

Obstructive and restrictive disorders characterize many medical chest diseases. Although these features are combined in many conditions, one of them usually predominates.

1 Obstructive disorders

The flow of air through the lungs may be reduced by obstruction in the airways. It can be assessed by measuring the forced expiratory volume in one second (FEV_1) which is normally 70–80% of the forced vital capacity (FVC) (fig. 44). The FEV_1 and FVC are recorded on machines which give a spirogram trace, such as the Vitalograph (fig. 45). Alternatively, the peak expiratory flow rate (PEFR) may be measured by means of the Wright Peak Flow Meter or the Mini–Wright Peak Flow Meter. These devices measure the maximum flow that can be maintained for 10 milliseconds at the beginning of expiration (figs. 46 & 47).

If the FEV_1 and PEFR improve following the administration of a bronchodilator the condition is recognized as *reversible airflow obstruction* (fig. 48). This is frequently seen in asthma and chronic bronchitis. Reversible airflow obstruction is caused by bronchospasm, oedema of the bronchial mucosa or excessive secretions and a combination of all 3 is often present.

If the FEV_1 and PEFR do not improve

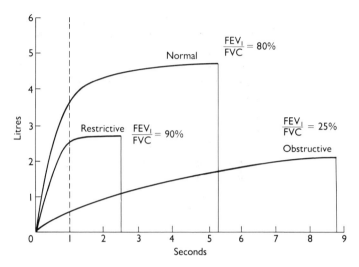

Fig. 44. *Spirometry in normal airways and obstructive and restrictive disorders.*

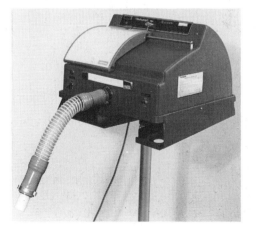

Fig. 45. *The Vitalograph.*

following the administration of a bronchodilator, this is known as *irreversible airflow obstruction*. It is a sign of structural damage of the airways and is seen in emphysema, severe chronic bronchitis and generalized bronchiectasis.

The patient may feel some relief after a

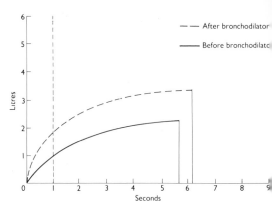

Fig. 48. *Spirometry showing reversibility of airways: increase in FEV$_1$ and FVC.*

bronchodilator and this may be due to very slight reversibility in the airflow obstruction which is shown by increase in FVC, although no change is registered in PEFR or FEV$_1$. This increase in FVC reflects the fact that some deflation of the overdistended lungs has occurred as a result of slight dilatation of the airways (fig. 49).

Peak flow meters are simple, portable devices useful to assess airflow obstruction where there is a considerable degree of reversibility, but with largely irrever-

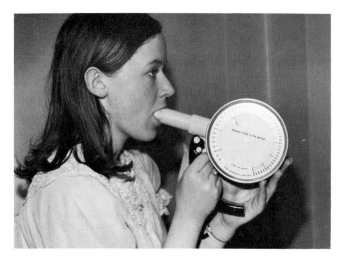

Fig. 46. *Wright Peak Flow Meter in use.*

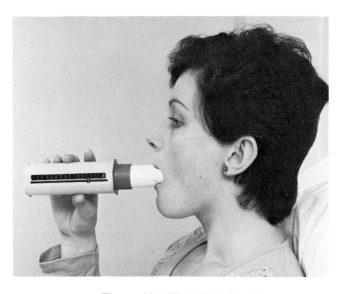

Fig. 47. *Mini–Wright Peak Flow Meter.*

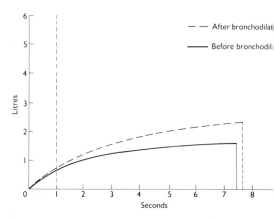

Fig. 49. *Spirometry showing an increase in FVC only.*

sible airways where minimal change is important, spirometry is more informative.

A patient's response to bronchodilator drugs can be accurately assessed by measurements of FEV_I and FVC. Bronchodilator drugs should not have been given for 4–6 hours preceding the test. This time will minimize the effect of drugs previously taken. Stable baseline readings, with correct technique, must first be obtained. The best result of two or three attempts is taken, allowing at least a 30 second pause between them. Baseline readings are repeated at 5 minute intervals until the maximum pre-treatment level is known. Some patients will continue to improve over several minutes while others will soon reach a plateau or decrease their FEV_I or FVC.

Having ensured a correct technique the bronchodilator is then inhaled and spirometry is repeated at the appropriate time interval for the particular drug. After salbutamol (Ventolin), or terbutaline (Bricanyl), readings can be made at 15- and 30-minute intervals (Ruffin et al. 1977), whereas with the slower acting ipratropium bromide (Atrovent), recordings are made 40 and 60 minutes from the time of inhalation (Loddenkemper 1975). In each case recordings should be continued until the maximum response is achieved, for example if the response to salbutamol is greater at 30 minutes than at 15 minutes, the spirometry is repeated at 10-minute intervals until a plateau or fall in FEV_I or FVC is recorded. If time is limited, this outline can be modified, recordings being taken at the expected times of maximal improvement (30 minutes following Ventolin and Bricanyl and 60 minutes following Atrovent).

The same principle can be applied when comparing different methods of delivery of the same drug or when comparing the response to two different bronchodilators. If comparing the response of a patient to Ventolin by pressurized aerosol and a nebulized solution of Ventolin, measurements are made until maximum response is reached after inhalation by pressurized aerosol and then the nebulized solution is given immediately. Any additional response is determined by the post-nebulizer recordings. If response to one method of delivery is determined on one occasion and to the other method on a separate occasion, it is impossible to compare the results accurately because the baseline readings and other factors such as the time of testing and dose of steroid drugs may be different.

Similarly when comparing the response to two different drugs (for example Ventolin and Atrovent) the second should be given as soon as maximum response has been achieved with the first.

2 Restrictive disorders

Pulmonary expansion may be restricted by abnormalities of the rib cage, pleura or lungs.

Disorders of the rib cage include conditions such as ankylosing spondylitis and kyphoscoliosis. The flow of air in the lungs is reduced although there is no disease.

With disorders of the pleura or lungs, such as pleural fibrosis, interstitial pulmonary fibrosis (fibrosing alveolitis) or pulmonary oedema, there is a decrease in pulmonary compliance (increased stiffness) which restricts lung expansion.

The lung volumes are reduced in patients with restrictive lung disease

43

(fig. 44) and to achieve adequate gaseous exchange breathing may be rapid (tachypnoea).

Diseases of the lung itself often interfere with the alveolar wall adding difficulties of gas transfer to those of pulmonary restriction.

ASSESSMENT OF THE PATIENT

Before starting treatment, the physiotherapist should assess the condition of the patient. Important facts are ascertained by reading the medical history, looking at chest radiographs and their reports, as well as reports of relevant investigations such as lung function tests, blood gases and bacteriology.

Brief clinical examination of the patient, observation and simple questioning will provide further information. The following are some questions that the physiotherapist should consider:

1 Relevant *history* of the illness.

2 *Exercise tolerance*. Is the patient short of breath (dyspnoeic) at rest or only on exertion? Has it prevented him from working? How far can he walk in 6 minutes? (p. 51). Does he get short of breath walking upstairs?

3 *Breathing pattern*. Is the thorax held in an overinflated position? Are the accessory muscles of respiration being overworked? Is there any deformity or obvious restriction of movement? When a deep breath is taken, is there a sudden 'catch' in breathing due to pleuritic pain? What is the rate of breathing? Is there equal expansion of both sides of the lower rib cage? Is there paradoxical movement of the chest wall? Is there tracheal tug (the larynx descending with each inspiration probably caused by pull from a low flattened diaphragm)? Chest measurements can be taken if no other means of assessment is available, but cannot be reproduced with accuracy. They are taken at full inspiration, full expiration and in the resting position, at three levels:

(a) in the axilla at the level of the 4th rib

(b) in the epigastric region at the level of the 9th costal cartilage

(c) in the subcostal region with the tape measure below the ribs.

4 *Breath sounds*. Auscultation (p. 13) may be helpful, but valuable information such as the presence of wheeze, stridor or crackles can be acquired by listening to the patient's breathing and coughing without a stethoscope.

5 *Cough*. Is the cough productive or nonproductive? Does the cough sound effective?

6 *Sputum*. What volume is produced daily? Is it mucoid (clear or white), mucopurulent, purulent (infected), rusty (typical of lobar pneumonia), blood stained (p. 30), or does it contain plugs or casts (typical of some cases of asthma and bronchopulmonary aspergillosis (p. 71))?

7 *Chest pain*. Is there pain due to the pulmonary condition such as pleuritic pain? Is there skeletal pain due to osteoporosis or metastatic disease? Is it due to myocardial insufficiency?

8 *Oedema*. Are the feet and ankles oedematous?

9 *Colour*. Is the patient cyanosed?

10 *Hands*. Are the fingers clubbed?

11 *Airflow obstruction*. What are the FEV_1 and FVC, or PEFR? Where simple lung function tests have previously been recorded, repeating the tests will enable comparisons to be made giving an indication of the severity and nature of the

condition. They also provide an assessment of the degree of reversibility which may be expected as a result of treatment.

OBSTRUCTIVE DISORDERS

This group of disorders includes chronic bronchitis, emphysema and asthma.

CHRONIC BRONCHITIS AND EMPHYSEMA

Chronic bronchitis has been defined (World Health Organization 1961) as a condition in which there is a chronic or recurrent increase above the normal in the volume of bronchial mucus secretion, sufficient to cause expectoration, when this condition is not due to localized bronchopulmonary disease. The words 'chronic' or 'recurrent' may be further defined as when the cough is present on most days during at least 3 months in each of 2 successive years.

A later definition (Medical Research Council 1965) subdivided chronic bronchitis into simple chronic bronchitis, chronic or recurrent mucopurulent bronchitis and chronic obstructive bronchitis.

Emphysema is a condition in which there is increase beyond the normal in the size of air spaces distal to the terminal bronchiole, with destructive changes in their walls (World Health Organization 1961).

More recently it has been shown that there are two distinct disorders, obstructive and hypersecretory. These commonly occur together, but may develop independently (Fletcher *et al.* 1976). With the hypersecretory disorder there is hypertrophy of the mucus secreting glands in the bronchial walls and an increase in goblet cells in the epithelial lining of the bronchial tree causing expectoration and a predisposition to bronchial infection. The obstructive disorder causes impairment of expiratory flow leading to eventual disability.

Many patients have a combination of these disorders and repeated infections may damage the alveoli with acute inflammation and their weakened walls may rupture. The bronchioles become scarred and distorted and on expiration air trapping occurs. Cigarette smoking is a major factor in the development of both the hypersecretory and obstructive disorders and patients should be urged to stop.

If hypersecretion alone is present there will be a chronic productive cough without noticeable dyspnoea. There are usually no radiological changes of emphysema and the diffusing capacity of the lungs is normal. In the more advanced stage of the disease hypercapnia (a raised $Pa\text{CO}_2$) is common, the patient is cyanosed and cor pulmonale develops. These patients are sometimes known as 'blue bloaters'.

The signs and symptoms of patients with predominantly an obstructive disorder are dyspnoea usually with wheeze, a reduced FEV_1 with little or no response to a bronchodilator showing that there is largely irreversible airflow obstruction. With progression of the disease the patient becomes breathless at rest, increases the use of the accessory muscles of respiration and develops over-inflation of the upper chest with paradoxical indrawing of the lower rib cage on inspiration owing to the pull of the low flattened diaphragm. When radiological evidence of emphysema is present there will be a low flattened diaphragm, a large retrosternal air space and the heart may appear as a narrow vertical shadow. Bullae may be visible. In addition to a severe obstructive defect, pulmonary function tests show an increase in total lung capacity and residual volume and the ratio of the residual volume to total lung capacity is raised indicating air trapping. The diffusing capacity of the lungs is impaired. These patients, sometimes known as 'pink puffers', maintain a normal or low level of arterial carbon dioxide by hyperventilating in an effort to obtain an adequate arterial oxygen level. Cardiac failure does not develop until the terminal stage of the disease.

Many patients have both the hypersecretory and obstructive disorders in varying proportions leading to a mixture of signs and symptoms.

A minority of patients with emphysema may have the condition known as 'primary emphysema' which develops without any previous history of chest disease and is commonly associated with a familial deficiency in alpha$_1$-antitrypsin. Sputum production is unusual in these cases unless there is superimposed infection. The alveolar walls may disintegrate over a relatively short period leading to terminal respiratory failure.

Aims of treatment

1 To remove excess bronchial secretions and reduce airflow obstruction.
2 To reduce the work of breathing.
3 To teach control of breathing.
4 To mobilize the thorax.
5 To increase the patient's exercise tolerance.

1 Removal of excess bronchial secretions and reduction of airflow obstruction

All patients with chronic bronchitis should carry out regular postural drainage during the productive phases of their disease (p. 26). When secretions are minimal it may be sufficient to use the breathing techniques to clear secretions, in the sitting position alone. In the absence of infection the secretions are mucoid. Mucoid secretions are often small in volume, but clearance may require considerable effort on the part of the patient. Purulent secretions associated with infection tend to be larger in volume, but the patient may be able to expectorate more easily. The patient should be advised to note the colour of his secretions and be aware that antibiotics may be required if infection occurs.

In patients with 'primary emphysema' secretions are usually absent, but during an infective episode sputum may be present and postural drainage is indicated. In some patients with chronic bronchitis where emphysema is predominant, tipping may aggravate dyspnoea and postural drainage may need to be modified (p. 29).

Chest shaking should not be over-vigorous if the patient has been on high maintenance doses of corticosteroids as there is a tendency to osteoporosis and rib or vertebral fractures may result.

If the patient is unable to clear his chest adequately, it may be helpful to provide increased ventilation and humidification by means of intermittent positive pressure breathing (IPPB). This, in conjunction with postural drainage, will facilitate expectoration (p. 120).

There is often an element of broncho-

46

spasm associated with these disorders. If reversible bronchospasm is present, a bronchodilator may be given before postural drainage with IPPB, a nebulizer (p. 133) or a pressurized aerosol (p. 58). IPPB should not be used in the presence of emphysematous bullae because of the risk of causing a pneumothorax. It may be necessary to power the nebulizer from an air source if the patient is hypercapnic.

Spirometry before and after inhalation of a bronchodilator will indicate the degree of reversibility in the airways (p. 41). Some patients with obstructive disorders demonstrate a bronchodilator response to Ventolin. Atrovent has been shown to benefit some patients who do not respond to Ventolin alone and others demonstrate reversibility to Ventolin and Atrovent given together (Lightbody et al. 1978). In chronic bronchitis, Ventolin has been shown to increase the rate of mucociliary clearance (Lafortuna & Fazio 1984).

2 Breathing control and reduction of the work of breathing

During an attack of dyspnoea, the patient with bronchitis and/or emphysema tends to hold his chest in a position of inspiration. There is overactivity of the accessory muscles and diaphragmatic movement is inhibited. In severe emphysema there is often paradoxical movement of the chest wall, the lower ribs being drawn in on inspiration.

The pattern of breathing developed by an emphysematous patient is a short uncontrolled inspiration with increased use of the accessory muscles, followed by a prolonged and often forced expiration. This forced expiration produces a rise in intrathoracic pressure which may cause closure of the airways that are either damaged or no longer have the support of normal elastic lung tissue (fig. 50). This uncontrolled pattern of breathing is an exhausting and uneconomical method of ventilation, which the physiotherapist should attempt to reverse.

Some emphysematous patients spontaneously develop a technique of 'pursed-lip' breathing. These patients breathe out through the mouth with the lips held together loosely in a pursed position. It is possible that this improves respiration by increasing the end expiratory pressure. This method of breathing should not be discouraged, provided that it is carried out in a relaxed manner. If an attempt is made to teach this form of breathing to a patient who has not developed it spontaneously, there is a great danger of expiration

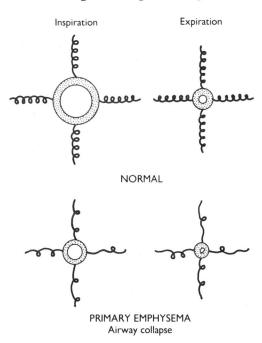

Fig. 50. *Airway collapse. By courtesy of Professor Lynne Reid.*

becoming forced, thus defeating the purpose of the technique. Unless this pattern is already established, it should be omitted from the treatment programme.

All patients with obstructive disorders are taught to breathe with an active inspiratory phase using the lower chest and a passive, relaxed expiratory phase. If the patient can control his breathing, it can be of benefit during attacks of dyspnoea. The rest positions (figs 51–56) encourage maximal relaxation of the upper chest and freedom of movement of the lower chest. They can be adapted to different situations in everyday life. At this stage the rate of breathing is not important, but relaxation of the upper chest should be encouraged. The patient may prefer to breathe with his mouth open during an attack of dyspnoea. He should try to breathe gently using the lower chest without prolonging expiration (p. 16). When control of breathing has been achieved an effort should be made to slow down the respiratory rate.

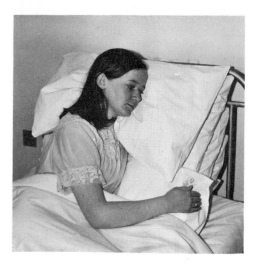

Fig. 51. *High side-lying.*

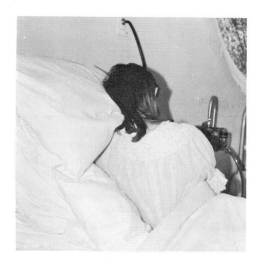

Fig. 52. *High side-lying (posterior aspect).*

HIGH SIDE-LYING (figs 51 & 52)

The patient lies on one side, slightly rolled forward, with a slope of three or four pillows to raise the shoulders and an extra pillow placed to fill the gap between the waist and axilla to prevent him sliding down the bed and to maintain a straight thoracic spine. The top pillow should be above the shoulder supporting only the head and neck. The underneath forearm can be placed either under the head pillow or resting on the bed under the pillow at the waist. The knees are slightly bent and the top leg placed in front of the lower one. This position is helpful for patients in acute respiratory distress, or at night for those suffering from orthopnoea.

FORWARD LEAN SITTING (fig. 53)

Many patients find this position comfortable. Two or three pillows are placed on a table and the patient can relax with the upper chest and head resting against them. The patient should maintain a

48

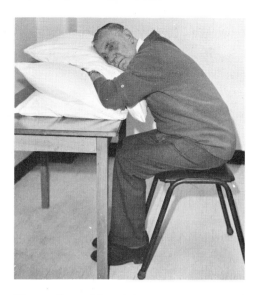

Fig. 53. *Forward lean sitting.*

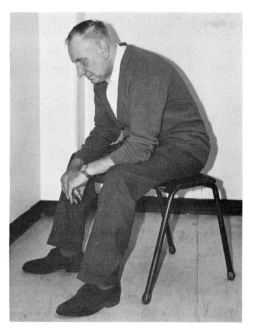

Fig. 54. *Relaxed sitting.*

straight thoracic and lumbar spine to avoid inhibiting lower chest movement.

RELAXED SITTING (fig. 54)

This is a useful position and can be taken up unobtrusively in public places. Many patients are inclined to grip their knees and raise their shoulders when in distress, but if they can sit leaning forward with the forearms resting on the thighs and the wrists relaxed, they will recover more quickly. If there is still a tendency to put pressure on the hands and forearms, some patients find relaxation easier with the forearms supinated and palms upwards. Care must be taken to ensure that the lumbar spine is not flexed, as this could impede free forward movement of the abdominal wall.

Obese patients will find it easier to lean back in a chair while relaxing their upper chest, forearms and hands. Their hands rest on the thighs.

FORWARD LEAN STANDING (fig. 55)

If there is nowhere to sit, distressed patients are inclined to grasp the nearest available object and hold themselves in a tense position. They should be encouraged to lean forward with the forearms resting on an object of suitable height.

RELAXED STANDING (fig. 56)

The distressed patient may also gain relief by leaning back against a wall or upright support. The feet should be approximately 30 cm from the wall, the shoulders relaxed and arms hanging by the sides. Alternatively he may lean sideways against a support.

49

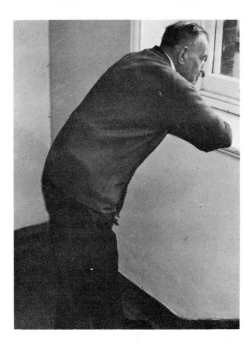

Fig. 55. *Forward lean standing.*

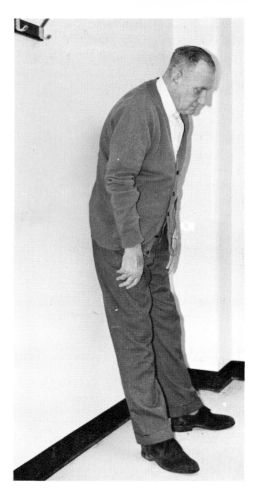

Fig. 56. *Relaxed standing.*

CONTROL OF BREATHING DURING EXERCISE

When the patient is able to control his breathing in these relaxed positions he should practise while sitting and standing upright without support. Progression can then be made to control of breathing while walking on the level, on stairs and on hills. Many patients tend to hold their breath during exercise. Breathing in rhythm with their steps can be helpful for example, breathing out for two steps and in for one step or out for one step and in for one step. It is often easier to teach patients using the 'one step in, one step out' pattern and this can be changed to another pattern if it is more suitable. A breathing pattern must be established for each individual and be altered as necessary under differing circumstances.

Some patients tend to become distressed when bending forward (for example to tie shoe laces). Many of them breathe in before bending down and experience discomfort due to the upward pressure of the abdominal contents against the flattened diaphragm. This discomfort is less if breathing out is encouraged whilst bending down. Breathing in takes place during the return to an upright position.

Although pulmonary function tests do not show any significant improvements in patients who have been taught breathing control (Grant 1970) they appear to derive benefit from the fact that they are breathing in a more economical manner. By eliminating unnecessary muscle activity during respiration, the work of breathing is reduced. Subjective improvement in ability to carry out daily living activities has been obtained using control of breathing (Booker *et al.* 1985).

3 Mobilization of the thorax

Treatment is not progressed until the patient has mastered breathing control and relaxation of the upper chest both during and between attacks of dyspnoea.

Thoracic expansion exercises (p. 17) are then started. By improving the mobility of the lower thoracic cage together with relaxation of the upper chest, the patient should achieve a more normal pattern of breathing.

In patients with emphysema, the domes of the diaphragm are flattened or even inverted. This abnormal position of the diaphragm can cause rib retraction on inspiration, but with perseverance a little lateral basal movement may be achieved (Hooper 1967).

4 Increase of exercise tolerance

There is a poor correlation between lung function and exercise ability. Some patients with severe airflow obstruction are able to work and walk without distress, while others with less severe airflow obstruction lead very restricted lives as a result of the feeling of breathlessness.

The aim of physiotherapy for severely disabled patients is to increase their exercise tolerance to enable them to carry out useful daily activities and improve their quality of life. Patients should be encouraged to be as mobile and active as possible. Their exercise tolerance may be increased by gradually increasing the distances walked, both on the level and on slopes and stairs, while practising breathing control.

The 6-minute walking test is a simple and reproducible method of assessing the exercise ability of the chronic breathless patient. The test originally described was a 12-minute walking test (McGavin *et al.* 1976a), but a 6-minute test has been shown to correlate well with the 12-minute test (Butland *et al.* 1982) and is more convenient. It is described as the greatest distance that the subject can walk in 6 minutes in a level enclosed corridor, regardless of whether or not he has to stop for rest.

The patient is instructed to walk up and down the corridor as many times as he can in the 6 minutes and is told that by the end of the test he should feel that he could not have managed any further distance. A few patients may need to stop and rest during the test and this time is included in the 6 minutes.

It is a self-paced test and therefore essential that the patient walks on his own, with the physiotherapist giving him encouragement and telling him the time at intervals.

At least one practice 6-minute walk is necessary before the results are reproducible. If the practice test is carried out within a day or two of the next test there is no need to do more than one practice, but if a longer period elapses two practice walks are necessary as shown in a study where walks were performed at monthly intervals (Mungall & Hainsworth 1979). The test is helpful in assessment before beginning an exercise programme and to determine progress.

Visual analogue scales (VAS) have been found to be a useful method of quantifying breathlessness (Woodcock et al. 1981). The patient scores the severity of breathlessness on a 10 cm line marked 'not breathless' at one end and 'extremely breathless' at the other. A combination of the 6-minute walking test and VAS can be used to assess the benefit of portable oxygen to very disabled patients. Portable cylinders containing air or oxygen are used with the patient unaware of the contents. Three walks are undertaken with a rest period of at least 30 minutes between walks. The first walk is a practice walk and is followed by two test walks using compressed air and oxygen in random order. Oxygen has been found to reduce the sensation of breathlessness and increase the distance walked in some patients (Waterhouse & Howard 1983). An alternative method of studying the effect of portable oxygen on exercise ability is by measuring arterial oxygen saturation (Brambilla et al. 1987).

A simple graduated exercise scheme has been shown to increase exercise tolerance as judged by the 12-minute walking test, while ventilatory function tests remained unchanged (McGavin et al. 1977). An exercise scheme for patients to carry out at home, starts with the daily climbing of five steps for 2 minutes and week by week the number of steps or minutes is gradually increased. The aim is to build up to climbing ten steps for 10 minutes at least once daily. If no staircase is available, a similar scheme can be devised walking on the level. For either of these exercise programmes it is important that the patient keeps a daily record card of his achievements. The patient must understand that during the exercise programme and 6-minute walking test he is expected to become breathless, but at all other times his aim should be to walk on the level, slopes or stairs using breathing control to minimize breathlessness.

Some severely emphysematous patients are unable to make any progress with a stair climbing programme (Booker et al. 1985). These patients derive more benefit by walking increasing distances using breathing control.

Contra-indications to the exercise scheme include interstitial lung disease, for example diffuse fibrosing alveolitis, malignant pulmonary and pleural diseases, ischaemic heart disease and intermittent claudication.

There are differing views on the physiological changes in heart rate and oxygen uptake produced by exercise training of the chronic bronchitic (McGavin et al. 1977), but the most likely physiological explanation for improvement concerns the oxygen cost of exercise. With training the activity is performed more efficiently and requires less oxygen. There is also a psychological component in improved exercise tolerance. Fear is reduced once the patient is persuaded that breathlessness is uncomfortable but not harmful. Training helps him to gain confidence and often increases tolerance to the sensation of breathlessness.

In some hospitals a graduated training programme using a treadmill or bicycle ergometer is used, but it seems more appropriate to provide a programme that can be carried out in the home and has the effect of training for an activity related to daily life.

Inhalation of a bronchodilator preceding exercise can improve exercise tolerance, although the extent of the improvement does not correlate with changes in FEV_1 or FVC (McGavin *et al.* 1976b).

A few patients are so disabled that they need a respiratory walking frame to walk even a short distance (fig. 57). A portable oxygen cylinder can be attached to the frame if necessary.

Opinions differ regarding the use of inspiratory muscle training for patients with chronic bronchitis and emphysema. It has been suggested that fatigue of the respiratory muscles may contribute to respiratory failure and attempts have been made to train these muscles in the hope that the onset of respiratory failure may be delayed.

The patient breathes through a mouthpiece or facemask with a resistance applied to the inspiratory limb of a valve. By changing the size of the inspiratory orifice, the resistance can be altered while the expiratory limb remains unimpeded. The exercise programme varies according to whether emphasis is being placed on endurance or muscle strength.

Many small studies, some performed without control groups, have investigated inspiratory muscle training and have led to conflicting evidence. A large-scale controlled study may yield evidence of benefit from inspiratory muscle training, but it is considered that the benefit is likely to be small (Flenley 1985).

In many patients with chronic bronchitis and emphysema the diaphragm is flattened, the chest is hyperinflated and the muscles of respiration not only work at a mechanical disadvantage, but are overworked. It is possible that these muscles are already 'trained'.

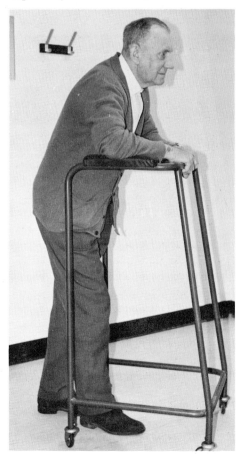

Fig. 57. *Respiratory walking frame.*

Home instruction

It is essential that all patients with chronic airflow limitation continue physiotherapy at home. Instruction leaflets and exercise record cards are helpful. Prolonged outpatient treatment is unnecessary if careful instructions have been given.

Acute exacerbation of chronic bronchitis

If a patient with chronic bronchitis develops an acute infection, his condition may deteriorate rapidly. Excess bronchial secretion is produced and although some is expectorated, a considerable quantity remains in the bronchial tree contributing to airflow obstruction. Swelling of the bronchial mucosa due to the infection will decrease the lumen of the air passages and further contribute to obstruction. This obstruction to ventilation results in inadequate gas exchange in the periphery of the lung. The Pao$_2$ falls while the Paco$_2$ rises. As a result, the patient becomes drowsy and confused and his breathing becomes erratic, shallow and inefficient.

At this stage, vigorous physiotherapy is essential. The usual methods of postural drainage may not be effective because the patient may be unable to cooperate with breathing exercises, huffing and coughing. IPPB can be of great value here and may obviate the need for intubation (p. 125). Assisted ventilation with vigorous chest shaking and postural drainage, as tolerated, aerates the lungs more effectively and loosens secretions. The patient often begins to cough spontaneously and becomes more alert. During the early, acute stage of the exacerbation it may be necessary to repeat the treatment at hourly intervals.

Dehydration is often a problem in the acute stage making expectoration of viscid secretions difficult. Encouraging the patient to take frequent drinks will help, together with humidification of the inspired gases. A venturi mask providing controlled oxygen therapy is usually required and to humidify such a mask adequately, a humidity adapter is useful (p. 137).

Cor pulmonale

Cor pulmonale has been defined as:

'Hypertrophy of the right ventricle resulting from diseases affecting the function and/or structure of the lung, except when these pulmonary alterations are the result of diseases that primarily affect the left side of the heart or of congenital heart disease' (World Health Organization 1961).

Cor pulmonale most commonly occurs in association with longstanding pulmonary disease such as chronic bronchitis or bronchiectasis. It is also seen in patients with kyphoscoliosis. It rarely occurs in primary emphysema.

A respiratory infection superimposed on one of these conditions frequently precipitates cor pulmonale. The respiratory infection causes carbon dioxide retention and hypoxia and these together cause constriction of the pulmonary arterioles so producing pulmonary hypertension. Many pulmonary blood vessels are obliterated by disease of lung tissue making the passage of blood through the pulmonary circulation even more difficult. A radiograph of the chest will show cardiac enlargement and dilatation of the main pulmonary arteries. In the later stages of cor pulmonale, right ventricular failure develops due to the enormous work load and continuing hypoxia.

Physiotherapy is required to clear excess secretions and to improve alveolar ventilation. Other treatment includes oxygen therapy, antibiotics and diuretics. It must be understood that the right-sided heart failure in cor pulmonale will not be relieved until the chest condition has been treated.

An alternative method of treatment of cor pulmonale is negative pressure ventilation by means of a tank ventilator (Mosley 1985). It has been found useful in correcting alveolar hypoventilation in disorders of the chest wall such as kyphoscoliosis or previous thoracoplasty. This means of mechanical ventilation is non-invasive and can be used instead of intubation and ventilation by intermittent positive pressure (IPPV). The difficult weaning phase of the chronic respiratory patient is avoided. Disadvantages of the tank ventilator and other negative pressure ventilators, for example a cuirasse or pneumosuit, are that they are cumbersome and difficult for the patient to apply. Nasal IPPV may be used increasingly in the future.

Tank respirators were originally designed for paralysed patients and physiotherapy to assist clearance of secretions can be given effectively with the patient in the respirator. Manual chest compression and assisted coughing are given by placing the hands through the portholes of the respirator (Higgens 1966). Patients who are not paralysed and have an effective cough may be more comfortably and effectively treated out of the tank respirator, on a bed. IPPB is often useful to assist loosening of secretions (p. 120).

Respiratory failure during sleep

Some patients with a restrictive or obstructive pulmonary disorder develop severe respiratory failure during sleep and require some means of improving ventilation.

Protriptyline is a drug which reduces the amount of rapid eye movement (REM) sleep. It is during this stage of sleep that severe hypoxia can occur and reduction of this sleep pattern often gives sufficient benefit to prevent respiratory failure (Simonds et al. 1986a).

Negative pressure ventilation has been used for some patients, but one disadvantage is that upper airway obstruction can occur during sleep in a tank ventilator and with the other forms of negative pressure ventilation. Positive pressure ventilation by nasal mask is being investigated in this group of patients (Carroll & Branthwaite 1987).

Positive pressure ventilation by nasal mask has been shown to prevent nocturnal hypoxaemia and hypercapnia in patients with neuromuscular disease. During negative pressure ventilation in these patients, upper airway obstruction occurred during REM sleep and was not a satisfactory method of eliminating respiratory failure (Ellis et al. 1987).

ASTHMA

Asthma is defined as narrowing of the airways which varies over short periods of time either spontaneously or as a result of treatment.

Asthmatic patients may be classified as being atopic or non-atopic. Atopic subjects have raised serum levels of total IgE antibody, with specific IgE antibody to allergens such as grass pollen and house dust mites and have positive immediate skin prick test reactions elicited by such allergens. Symptoms often start in infancy with flexural eczema, followed by rhinitis and asthma provoked by exposure to specific allergens. There is often a family history of eczema, hay fever and asthma.

IgE antibody fixes to mast cells in the skin, eyes, nose and airways. Reaction of IgE on the surface of the mast cell with specific antigen such as grass pollen leads to the release of mediators, such as histamine, from the cell which cause local swelling in the skin (weal and flare reaction) and smooth muscle contraction (narrowing of the airways).

Non-atopic subjects do not have elevated total IgE levels in their serum. Skin tests with allergens such as grass pollen and house dust mites are negative and no specific IgE antibody to such allergens is found in their serum. Their asthma generally starts in adult life. They have not usually had eczema or hay fever and do not generally give a family history of these, although they may have a family history of asthma.

Both atopics and non-atopics may have asthmatic reactions provoked by specific or non-specific agents. Specific agents include occupational agents (such as toluene di-isocyanate and platinum salts) and drugs (such as aspirin and propranolol). Non-specific factors provoking asthma include upper respiratory tract infections, emotional upsets, exercise and inhalation of cold air.

Where provoking factors can be identified in either atopic or non-atopic individuals there is the possibility of finding effective treatment whether by removing the cause (occupational agent or known allergen), desensitizing the patient, or giving an appropriate prophylactic drug such as sodium cromoglycate (Intal) before exercise or exposure to the provoking stimulus.

Patients with intermittent asthmatic attacks will probably require regular bronchodilators and sodium cromoglycate, and those with persistent airway narrowing may also require long-term inhaled or oral corticosteroid treatment.

The narrowing of the airways in asthma is caused by a combination of three factors, bronchospasm (smooth muscle contraction), oedema of the mucus membrane and plugging with tenacious exudate. On admission to hospital with an acute, severe attack of asthma the patient is likely to be in respiratory distress with increased use of the accessory muscles of respiration. Wheeze is often audible, but in very severe cases there may be no wheeze owing to hyperinflation and a marked reduction in air flow. Wheeze, or lack of wheeze, is therefore not a satisfactory indication of severity of acute asthma.

Assessment of the severity of an attack is made by measurement of airflow obstruction (FEV_1 or PEFR), arterial blood gas levels, pulse rate and the degree of arterial paradox (pulsus paradoxus). As airflow obstruction increases, the arterial carbon dioxide level at first falls, but may gradually rise as the patient becomes exhausted. The arterial oxygen levels although low, is of less value in assessing the severity of asthma. Tachycardia is a feature of acute severe asthma. There may be a marked degree of arterial paradox which reflects abnormal intrathoracic pressures produced by airflow obstruction. Normally there is a fall in systolic blood pressure of up to 10 mmHg during inspiration, but levels of up to 40 mmHg may be present in a severe asthmatic attack. Increasing asthma also affects the electrocardiograph recording and changes suggesting acute pulmonary hypertension may be seen.

Drug and oxygen therapy are instituted immediately after assessment of the patient. The drugs commonly used are an intravenous infusion of aminophylline and hydrocortisone, with the addition of inhaled beta-adrenergic bronchodilators (for example Ventolin or Bricanyl) and oral corticosteroids. Physiotherapy is usually requested soon after admission to hospital.

In rare cases where drug therapy is not controlling the asthmatic attack, in that the FEV_I is not improving and the arterial carbon dioxide level is rising as the patient becomes more exhausted, intubation and mechanical ventilation may be indicated (p. 115).

Physiotherapists treat patients with a widely varying degree of asthma, ranging from those with a severe attack to those who are almost symptom free.

Aims of physiotherapy

1 To relieve bronchospasm.
2 To encourage relaxation and breathing control.
3 To assist removal of secretions.
4 To improve the pattern of breathing.
5 To educate the patient.

1 Relief of bronchospasm

This is the most important aspect of the treatment as it will be impossible to mobilize the secretions until bronchodilatation has started. The physiotherapist should remember that coughing and postural drainage if inappropriately used, may aggravate bronchospasm.

Bronchodilator drugs are usually administered by a nebulizer. In acute asthma the patient may be hypoxic and it is important to power the nebulizer with oxygen. The patient should be in a comfortable position, either in high side-lying (p. 48) or sitting upright, well supported by pillows. He is encouraged to relax the upper chest and shoulder girdle and inhale using the lower chest (fig. 58).

Treatment may be repeated 4 hourly during the acute stage and is gradually reduced as the patient improves. Patients

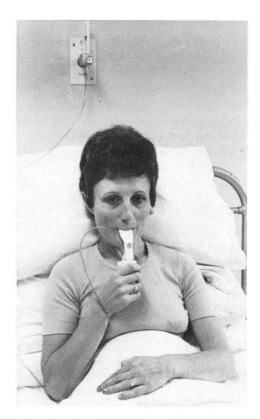

Fig. 58. *Inhalation from a nebulizer.*

who on awakening demonstrate a persistent fall in peak expiratory flow rate, or 'morning dip' (Turner–Warwick 1977), should not have the early morning treatment withdrawn until their condition stabilizes.

A few patients who are exhausted, benefit from the administration of the bronchodilator drugs by means of IPPB. When it is used correctly, the work of breathing is reduced while at the same time the drug is delivered (p. 126).

Simple lung function tests are carried out before and after treatment to assess the response to the bronchodilator (p. 41). A peak flow chart provides a useful record of the condition of asthmatic patients. On

57

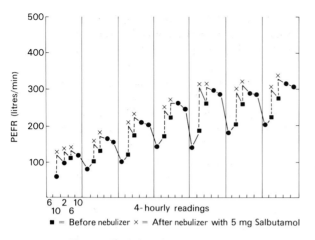

Fig. 59. *Peak flow chart.*

■ = Before nebulizer   × = After nebulizer with 5 mg Salbutamol

the chart shown (fig. 59) 4 hourly recordings have been made by the nursing staff from 6 am to 10 pm and the physiotherapist has recorded the peak expiratory flow rate before and 15 minutes after the completion of inhalation of a bronchodilator. It is often useful for the patient to monitor his condition objectively by using a peak flow meter at home.

The dosage of bronchodilator solution often prescribed in the treatment of asthma is 5 mg salbutamol (1 ml of 0·5% Ventolin respirator solution). When the patient starts to respond to other medical treatment a 2·5 mg dose is usually equally effective. Terbutaline has a similar action, the most common dose being 5 mg (0·5 ml of 1% Bricanyl respirator solution). The main side effect of these drugs is muscle tremor, especially of the hands. The physician will adjust the dosage of all bronchodilator drugs to reduce this to a minimum.

If bronchodilatation is not produced by beta-adrenergic drugs (salbutamol, terbutaline) an anticholinergic drug, such as ipratroprium bromide (Atrovent) may be prescribed. A dose of 0·25–0·5 mg (1–2 ml) of 0·025% Atrovent respirator solution is used and maximum response may not be reached until one hour after inhalation. Possible side effects are dryness of the mouth, retention of urine and dilation of the pupils with loss of visual accommodation. These effects are unlikely to occur with the normal therapeutic dose, but it is important to avoid Atrovent entering the eyes and therefore a mouthpiece, in preference to a face mask, should be used with a nebulizer. Atrovent has been shown to be an effective bronchodilator either alone or in combination with Ventolin (Lightbody et al. 1978).

As soon as a dry pressurized aerosol such as a Ventolin inhaler produces an equally good bronchodilator response, this should be used instead of the more expensive and complicated equipment required for nebulization. Instruction in the correct technique for using a pressurized aerosol is often necessary and before comparative tests of bronchodilator response (p. 43) are made, it is essential to ensure that the inhaler is being used correctly.

After shaking the pressurized aerosol (also known as a metered dose inhaler or MDI) the patient should exhale quietly and completely and having placed the aerosol up to the mouth, should press it firmly while inhaling slowly and deeply (fig. 60). To be effective it is important that the drug is released during the beginning of inspiration. After inhaling, the patient should hold his breath for a comfortable period of time (up to 10 seconds if possible) before breathing out quietly through the nose (Newman & Clarke 1983). A placebo inhaler is often helpful in teaching patients who are having difficulty in learning the technique

58

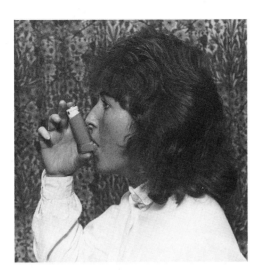

Fig. 60. *Inhaling from pressurized aerosol.*

and a modified aerosol incorporating a whistle can be useful (McGavin 1976).

For patients who have poor coordination and are unable to use a pressurized aerosol effectively, the Ventolin and Becotide Rotahalers have proved invaluable. This method of delivery is also useful for children and the elderly. Other devices to help those patients who have difficulty with coordination are the spacer tube and the valved spacer devices (fig. 61).

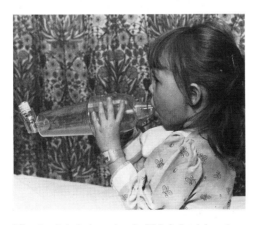

Fig. 61. *Inhalation using the Nebuhaler (Astra).*

In treatment of children it is essential that the appropriate device for inhalation is prescribed to suit the child's age and skill. Until 18 months of age inhalation therapy is usually possible only with a nebulizer. At this stage Atrovent is often more successful in bronchodilatation than the beta–adrenergic drugs (Ventolin and Bricanyl) possibly due to the immaturity of the beta receptors (Reiser & Warner 1986). Sodium cromoglycate may be used by nebulizer as a prophylactic drug.

From 18 months to 4 years some children can manage the valved spacer devices, but others may still need a nebulizer. The face mask is replaced by a mouthpiece as soon as the child can use one, to avoid deposition of the drug on the face and eyes and in the nose. From 4 to 8 years of age children can often manage the powder inhalers (rotahaler). These require minimal coordination and are less cumbersome and time consuming than nebulizer systems and valved spacers. In contrast to the technique for a pressurized aerosol, a faster inhalation with a rotahaler or spinhaler is necessary.

From about 8 years of age most children can coordinate sufficiently well to use a pressurized aerosol. A spacer tube does not appear to have any advantage when the aerosol is used efficiently, but it may be helpful in an acute attack when inhalation is difficult (Reiser & Warner 1986).

All patients using inhaled corticosteroid drugs (Becotide, Becloforte, Pulmicort) should be instructed to rinse their mouth out thoroughly after the inhalation to try and prevent candidiasis (thrush).

2 Relaxation and breathing control

Relaxation and breathing control are important in both severe and mild asthma.

The patient should be shown the relaxation positions described on p. 48–50, and encouraged to breathe gently using his lower chest at his own rate during attacks of dyspnoea. He should start to slow down his rate of breathing only when he has gained control. With sufficient practice breathing control, in conjunction with the prescribed drugs, can help during asthmatic attacks.

3 Removal of secretions

Great care must be taken not to aggravate bronchospasm when assisting with removal of secretions. If the patient's chest is too tight and wheezy to mobilize and expectorate secretions, the physiotherapist should not persist with this treatment, but wait until further bronchodilatation has taken place.

As soon as coughing results in the expectoration of sputum a modified form of postural drainage (p. 29) should be started. It has been shown that the forced expiration technique does not increase bronchospasm in asthmatic patients when used to aid clearance of bronchial secretions (Pryor & Webber 1979). The treatment should be given 10–15 minutes after administration of a bronchodilator. At this stage many patients start to expectorate thick, tenacious sputum which may contain casts. As the patient's condition improves, the foot of the bed can be tipped for postural drainage.

At the stage when secretions are thick and tenacious it may be of value to use IPPB for the mechanical assistance in mobilizing secretions. Heated humidity inhaled following bronchodilators may help loosen secretions, but care must be taken to ensure that bronchospasm is not aggravated (p. 138).

Many asthmatic patients have a productive cough between attacks and should include postural drainage in their home treatment. Inhalation of a bronchodilator if prescribed, should precede postural drainage.

4 Improvement of the breathing pattern

Lower thoracic expansion exercises should be started when there is improvement in the patient's condition. The patient should be made aware of his pattern of breathing and should be encouraged to relax the upper chest and minimize the action of the accessory muscles. It may be helpful to practice in front of a mirror, as many patients are unaware of their faulty pattern of breathing.

5 Education of the patient

The physiotherapist should be a member of the team involved in the education of the asthmatic patient about his condition and its management.

Exercise for asthmatics

Exercise may induce bronchoconstriction in asthmatic patients. It has been shown that there are significantly smaller falls in FEV_1 after swimming than after running and bicycling, (Fitch & Morton 1971) and it is now thought that the difference is probably due to different environmental conditions. Humidification or warming of the inspired air, as in a heated swimming pool, reduces exercise-induced asthma, whereas cooler air exacerbates the asthmatic response.

Evidence suggests that different types

of exercise produce similar degrees of exercise-induced asthma provided that ventilation and the environmental conditions are similar (Hartley 1979). It is thought that hyperventilation is probably the central mechanism in exercise-induced asthma, but it is not yet understood how hyperventilation and airway cooling lead to bronchoconstriction (Kilham *et al.* 1979).

Most children with asthma are able to participate in physical training at school provided that careful instruction has been given about prophylactic drugs to avoid exercise-induced asthma.

However, some children have not been allowed to participate at school and tend to develop poor posture, are unfit and lack confidence. They often avoid sports or exercise in their leisure time (Mallinson *et al.* 1981). These children benefit by physical training classes both physically and psycho-socially. Exercise classes include monitoring of PEFR or FEV_1, instruction in inhalation of drugs, warm-up exercises, progressive exercises for general strengthening and exercises to improve posture. Practise in coping with breathlessness and asthmatic attacks should also be included in a class.

Bronchitis and asthma in children

Recurrent 'chestiness' in children is a very common condition. Some children react to mild upper respiratory tract infections by coughing and wheezing and it may be difficult to make a clear distinction between bronchitis and asthma.

Infants and children respond well to postural drainage if they have excess secretions and from the age of 2 or 3 years it is possible to teach breathing exercises. The habit of mouth breathing should be discouraged and children need encouragement to blow their noses to clear the excess nasal secretions.

The principles of treatment are the same as for an adult, with modification of some positions as children are often comfortable lying flat during an attack of dyspnoea (figs 62–65). The inhalation of drugs and exercise for children with

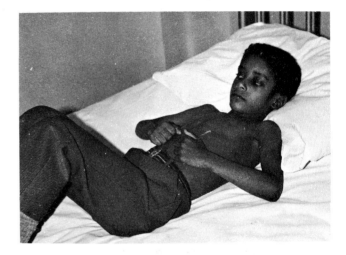

Fig. 62. *Breathing control.*

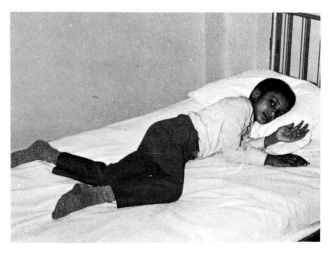

Fig. 63. *Breathing control.*

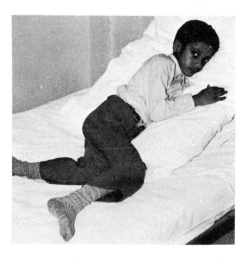

Fig. 64. *High side-lying for breathlessness.*

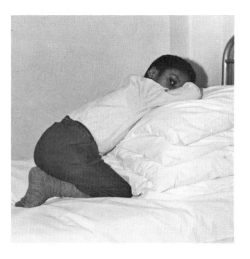

Fig. 65. *Kneeling position for breathlessness.*

asthma are discussed in the preceding section. Instructions should be given to parents in the supervision of breathing exercises and postural drainage at home and how to assist the child during wheezy episodes.

As children develop, the airways increase in size and the episodic narrowing of the airways may no longer be apparent.

PULMONARY INFECTIONS AND ASSOCIATED DISEASES

PNEUMONIA

Acute lobar pneumonia is not often seen in hospital as it responds quickly to antibiotic therapy if this is started in the early stages. If cases are admitted and physiotherapy is requested the treatment must not be confused with that appropriate for the more common bronchopneumonia.

Acute lobar pneumonia is characterized by fever, malaise and toxaemia. Pulmonary consolidation is present in one or more lobes and it is frequently due to infection by the pneumococcus. In the early stages of the disease the patient suffers from pleuritic pain, dyspnoea and a painful cough. Pleuritic pain is an acute localized chest pain, more marked on coughing or deep breathing and is due to inflammation of the pleura overlying the consolidated lobe. The cough is usually unproductive, but there may be scanty tenacious mucoid sputum, or it may be blood stained and 'rusty' in colour. An area of consolidation will be apparent on the radiograph. During this stage breathing exercises are encouraged. Chest shaking and percussion are not only painful, but of no benefit to the patient.

In the next stages of the disease, the pulmonary consolidation starts to resolve and as the pleuritic pain diminishes, coughing becomes less painful and sometimes productive of mucopurulent sputum. At this stage appropriate postural drainage is instituted and assistance given to clear secretions.

Bronchopneumonia, in contrast to lobar pneumonia, is patchy in distribution and is associated primarily with bronchial inflammatory change. It is seen more frequently than lobar pneumonia and commonly in post-operative patients, in chronic bronchitics and especially when these two situations co-exist. Physiotherapy is an essential part of the treatment regimen and is instituted immediately. Purulent or mucopurulent sputum is present in considerable quantities causing obstruction in the airways. As there is no consolidation or pleural inflammation causing pleuritic pain, there is no contra-indication to early physiotherapy. This consists of breathing techniques combined with postural drainage to assist the removal of secretions. If these measures are not effective, IPPB is used to assist ventilation and clearing of secretions (p. 120).

Mycoplasma pneumoniae is a common cause of pneumonia in previously healthy young people. Symptoms include mild fever and unproductive, persistent cough. Extensive patchy shadowing, usually unilateral, is seen on the radiograph. Instruction in breathing exercises may be given, but postural drainage is rarely necessary. The patient improves clinically, but the radiological changes may persist after discharge from hospital.

Legionnaire's disease is a severe form of pneumonia in which profound respiratory failure develops. Intermittent positive pressure ventilation (IPPV) may be required (p. 109). The radiograph shows patchy shadowing which is often unilateral. Sputum is usually minimal, but the physiotherapist should assess the patient and treat him according to his signs and symptoms.

LUNG ABSCESS

Postural drainage may be started as soon as a lung abscess is diagnosed. The abscess sometimes causes distortion of the bronchi and postural drainage positions may have to be modified to obtain effective drainage.

The use of IPPB is contra-indicated as there is a risk of causing air trapping in the cavity.

BRONCHIECTASIS

Bronchiectasis is characterized by dilatation of the bronchi associated with obstruction and infection. It can start in childhood following a respiratory infection such as pneumonia or whooping cough, or more rarely by obstruction of a bronchus as in primary tuberculosis (p. 68). Inhalation of a foreign body such as a peanut is another rare cause. Bronchiectasis occurs with cystic fibrosis, allergic bronchopulmonary aspergillosis (p. 71) and may complicate hypogammaglobulinaemia because of the patient's reduced capacity to resist bacterial infection. The diagnosis will be confirmed by a bronchogram.

Most patients have a productive cough with purulent sputum and suffer from repeated chest infections. Haemoptysis may occur in varying degrees and in some patients it may be their only symptom. This is known as 'dry' bronchiectasis.

Destruction of the cilia responsible for clearing the bronchi will have occurred as a result of the disease. Postural drainage is essential for patients with a productive cough. If the cilia survive, they may beat ineffectively due to the excessive secretions. These patients will have to continue postural drainage for the rest of their lives and instruction in home management is essential (p. 26).

Postural drainage is unnecessary for

patients with 'dry' bronchiectasis and it may aggravate the tendency to haemoptysis. If a mild haemoptysis occurs in productive patients, postural drainage may be continued. If severe haemoptysis occurs, physiotherapy should be discontinued temporarily until the bleeding has been controlled.

If the disease is sufficiently localized, surgery for removal of the affected lobe or lobes may be performed (p. 79).

CYSTIC FIBROSIS

Cystic fibrosis is a genetically determined disorder which has become increasingly recognized since it was first described by Andersen (1938). In this condition the exocrine glands are abnormal and the patients have an unusually high concentration of sodium in the sweat, abnormal pancreatic function and recurrent lung infections occur either together or separately. The abnormal pancreatic function results in malabsorption and steatorrhoea and the recurrent lung infections result in generalized suppurative bronchiectasis and the formation of multiple lung abscesses. The survival of these patients depends on the control of pulmonary infection and prevention of permanent lung damage. At one time it was unusual for these patients to survive over the age of 14, but with improved diagnosis and treatment many patients are now surviving to over the age of 40.

The introduction of postural drainage even before chest symptoms and signs have appeared is recommended by some physicians. This may delay the onset of chest complications and improve the overall prognosis. It should be remembered that radiological changes may be present without any detectable clinical change.

Treatment of the pulmonary complications consists of appropriate antibiotics and physiotherapy. Although antibiotic requirements may vary from time to time, physiotherapy must be a constant feature of the management even when the patient is apparently 'well'. During an exacerbation of the bronchopulmonary infection it is imperative that intensive physiotherapy is carried out. Even though the patient may attend a specialist hospital at intervals for follow up, the local hospital or domiciliary service should be prepared to offer facilities for physiotherapy if the patient and his relatives are unable to manage at home on these occasions.

The frequency and duration of *postural drainage* must be carefully assessed for each individual and the appropriate positions taught for the affected areas of the lungs. During an exacerbation the patient may need to spend as long as 20 minutes draining each area and it is often necessary to carry out treatment five times a day.

Often several lobes are affected and in order to give the patient some respite, the physiotherapist may have to be satisfied with treating two or three areas at one session and the other affected areas at the next session.

The home programme must be worked out for each individual. Many patients are able to treat themselves both effectively and efficiently without assistance, if instructed in postural drainage using the cycles of breathing techniques (p. 27, fig. 66). It has been shown that cystic fibrosis patients who have been relying on assistance with postural drainage at home can carry out their treatment more efficiently without assistance when using the active postural drainage cycle including the forced expiration technique (Pryor *et al.* 1979).

A portable, but stable tipping frame is an asset for many patients at home. A frame that supports the whole patient at an angle (fig. 67) is more comfortable and versatile than the frames that are angled at the centre which cannot support the patient comfortably for several of the required postural drainage positions.

Patients who produce sputum only occasionally should carry out postural drainage once a day, but those who produce sputum regularly should do it twice a day. If a patient has an upper respiratory tract infection, treatment must be carried out more frequently until the production of excess sputum has subsided. Postural drainage should not be done immediately following a meal and infants should be treated before their feeds. The most convenient times for treatment are usually early in the morning and in the evening either before going to bed or before going out to socialize.

Relatives of infants and small children should be instructed in the appropriate drainage positions and in the technique of clapping and vibratory-shaking. Until the child is able to walk, it is important to include drainage of the apical segments of the upper lobes as much of his time will be spent lying down.

In early childhood treatment has to be passive depending on clapping to stimulate coughing, but from about the age of 3 years the child should start to take an active part in the treatment using the cycle of breathing techniques (p. 27) in conjunction with the parent's clapping and shaking.

From the age of 9 or 10 years the child is usually ready to start learning to do his own treatment and can gradually become

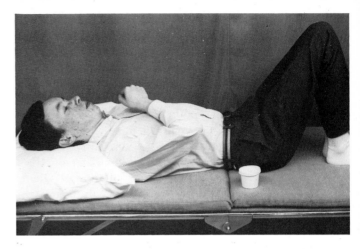

Fig. 66. *Self-postural drainage for the anterior segments of the upper lobes.*

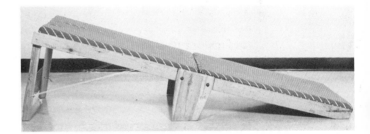

Fig. 67. *Postural drainage frame.*

independent of his parents' help. The techniques must be taught very carefully and it is helpful to let the parents watch while the child is treating himself under the physiotherapist's supervision. This gives the parents the confidence that their child is capable of independent treatment and will be able to manage satisfactorily when away from home.

Adolescents often become resentful of their condition and may rebel against treatment by their parents. If they have learnt to do their own postural drainage, this difficult period may be less problematic. The physiotherapist must emphasize

65

the importance of postural drainage and try and persuade him to do it.

After leaving school there may be a problem fitting in the treatment around the hours of work, but a solution must be worked out.

A physiotherapist should see all cystic fibrosis patients at regular intervals, for example when attending the doctor's follow-up clinic, in order to assess the chest condition, suggest any alterations in home treatment and discuss any problems that have arisen. It may occasionally be necessary to arrange domiciliary physiotherapy, but it is unlikely to be required on a long-term basis.

Breathing exercises are an integral part of postural drainage. Dyspnoeic patients are shown relaxation positions (p. 48) and are instructed in breathing control in these positions and when climbing stairs or hills.

With the development of an over-inflated upper chest and rigid lower rib cage, many patients tend to a kyphotic posture. Exercises to *mobilize the shoulder girdle and trunk* and to *correct posture* should be included in the treatment programme.

Exercise programmes that have been carried out by cystic fibrosis patients have increased fitness and exercise tolerance, although pulmonary function has not changed (Orenstein *et al.* 1983). It has also been shown that, with exercise training, the feeling of breathlessness is relieved and therefore exercise is better tolerated (O'Neill *et al.* 1987).

Exercise should be encouraged for all patients. Most children are able to participate in physical education at school and all patients will benefit from some form of exercise (fig. 68). Non-competitive sports may be more suitable and more enjoyable

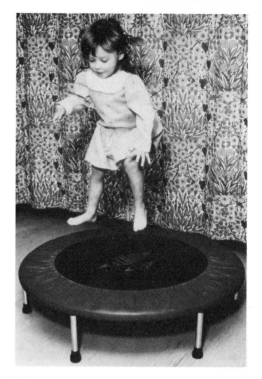

Fig. 68. *Enjoying a bounce.*

for the more severely affected patients. A stationary bicycle (fig. 69) is often useful to provide a progressive exercise programme in the winter period when outdoor sports are not appropriate.

In patients with minimal sputum, it is likely that exercise may be as beneficial as postural drainage, but for the majority of patients who regularly produce sputum it is advisable to do exercise in addition to postural drainage. Exercise will probably help to loosen secretions and the time of postural drainage may be shortened, but it should not be considered an alternative treatment.

In some countries the regular use of *mist tents* at night has been advocated, but it has been shown that mist tent therapy evaluated over a 6 month period had no

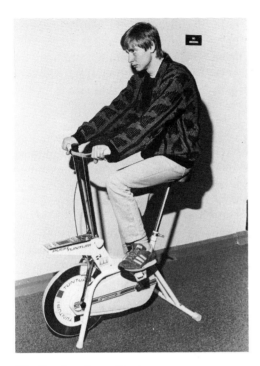

Fig. 69. *A stationary bicycle.*

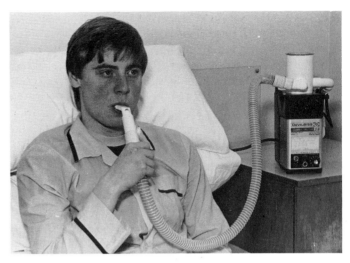

Fig. 70. *Humidification from an ultrasonic nebulizer (De Vilbiss).*

beneficial effect (Rosenbluth & Chernick 1974) and a further study has shown no decrease in sputum viscosity or enhancement of the removal of secretions (Chang *et al.* 1973). During an acute exacerbation of the bronchopulmonary infection, patients often find it easier to expectorate after inhaling mist from an efficient nebulizer by mouthpiece (fig. 70). If the patient is being nursed with an oxygen mask, high *humidification* should be incorporated into the system with wide bore tubing (p. 137).

Inhalation from a nebulizer powered by a suitable air compressor is useful for many patients at home. Small children need a face mask, but a mouthpiece provides more effective delivery of drugs and should be used when possible (p. 131).

Cystic fibrosis patients may have some reversibility in their airways and benefit from bronchodilator drugs preceding postural drainage. The inhalation of beta–adrenergic drugs (Ventolin and Bricanyl) has been shown to improve cilial action (Wood *et al.* 1975) and if no bronchodilator response is seen, one of these drugs may be beneficial in assisting mucociliary clearance.

Normal saline (0·9%), hypertonic saline (7%) or mucolytic drugs may be inhaled, before postural drainage, to assist clearance of secretions (p. 134). Mucolytic drugs may cause an irritant effect on the airways and should be used with caution (p. 30).

Carefully selected patients with persistent pseudomonas infection and deteriorating lung function often benefit from the inhalation of antibiotic drugs (Hodson *et al.* 1981). These are usually prescribed to be inhaled twice daily following postural drainage. Occasionally there is an increase in airflow obstruction with inhalation of some antibiotics. Spirometry should be

67

carried out before and after inhalation on the first occasion. Appropriate timing of a dose of bronchodilator drugs may avoid an increase in airflow obstruction. Provision of suitable equipment for inhalation of antibiotics is essential (p. 133).

IPPB and periodic continuous positive airway pressure (PCPAP) should be used with caution in the treatment of cystic fibrosis because there is the possibility of causing a pneumothorax and IPPB has also been shown to increase the residual volume in these patients after a prolonged period of treatment (Matthews *et al.* 1964). In patients with an acute exacerbation who have become exhausted and unable to clear their secretions adequately, IPPB has proved useful during postural drainage. Short periods of treatment, lasting a maximum of 14 days are recommended in these circumstances and the inspiratory pressure should be kept low (below 11 cmH$_2$O).

Complications of cystic fibrosis include haemoptysis and spontaneous pneumothorax. Many patients have occasional mild *haemoptyses*. If there is only slight streaking of the sputum, the postural drainage routine can be continued avoiding vigorous percussion. If a more severe haemoptysis occurs, percussion should be omitted until the bleeding decreases. Attempts should be made to avoid persistent coughing and use huffing gently to mobilize secretions as less intrathoracic pressure is created. Where very severe bleeding occurs, postural drainage should be temporarily discontinued, but resumed as soon as possible to remove any blood that has accumulated in the lungs.

If haemoptysis is severe and persistent, embolization of the bronchial artery may be carried out under radiological vision in an attempt to stop the bleeding. There is hypertrophy of the bronchial arteries in cystic fibrosis patients with advanced pulmonary disease. Gelatin foam is introduced by catheterization via the femoral artery (Batten & Matthew 1983). Following the procedure, physiotherapy can be resumed without delay.

Spontaneous pneumothorax can occur in the older patient. A small pneumothorax may absorb spontaneously and physiotherapy is continued. A larger pneumothorax may require an intercostal drainage tube, attached to an underwater seal and physiotherapy is discontinued until it has been inserted. Clapping should be avoided over the site of the tube. Analgesia may be helpful preceding treatment. Thoracic expansion exercises may be encouraged in between postural drainage sessions to assist re-expansion of the affected lung. If the air-leak persists, surgery, in the form of pleurodesis or pleurectomy, may be indicated (p. 95).

Physiotherapy should be continued during the *terminal stage* of the disease, even though it may achieve little physical improvement. Treatment will have become such an integral part of the patient's life that withdrawal at this stage would cause anxiety. The extent of treatment should be considered carefully and it should not be allowed to cause undue exhaustion. Nasopharyngeal suction should not be considered as it is an unpleasant procedure and would serve no useful purpose at this stage. Assessment for heart-lung transplantation is considered for some of these patients.

PULMONARY TUBERCULOSIS

Pulmonary tuberculosis has become less common since the improvement of public health standards and treatment by effective chemotherapy. Physiotherapy is rarely requested for this condition, but it is sometimes necessary to treat associated complications.

The first infection with the tubercle bacillus is known as *primary tuberculosis*. A small pneumonic lesion may occur in any part of the lung and the nearest lymph glands become enlarged. The lesion usually heals by fibrosis and calcification and subsequently causes no problem. Occasionally it spreads through the lobe and may then cavitate. If pleural effusion occurs, thoracic expansion exercises are required (p. 17).

In infants and young children the enlarged hilar lymph nodes may compress a bronchus and cause segmental collapse. Prolonged compression may lead to permanent bronchiectasis as in the '*middle lobe syndrome*'. Another cause of segmental collapse may be discharge of caseous material from the affected lymph gland into the bronchus. Physiotherapy may be requested to attempt re-expansion of a collapsed middle lobe. The result may be disappointing, but it is worth persevering with breathing exercises and postural drainage as re-expansion sometimes occurs.

Post-primary tuberculosis is a re-infection after the primary lesion. The infection usually occurs in the upper lobes or apical segments of the lower lobes. A small area of tuberculous bronchopneumonia appears at first and this spreads by direct infection to neighbouring lung tissue. Caseation follows and the necrotic centre of the lesion is discharged into a bronchus leaving a cavity. The patient coughs up infective sputum, some of which may be inhaled into other areas of lung producing new tuberculous lesions. Haemoptysis occurs if there is erosion of blood vessels.

Peripheral lesions may cause pleurisy leading to *tuberculous effusion* or *empyema*.

In these cases breathing exercises are important to prevent chest deformity and loss of respiratory function by pleural thickening (p. 74). There is no risk of these exercises causing spread of the disease once medical treatment has been established.

In contrast to acute tuberculosis with infiltration and cavitation, a *chronic fibro-caseous* condition may develop. Gross fibrous contraction of the upper lobes with compensatory emphysema of the lower lobes results in dyspnoea and diminished respiratory reserve. Assistance with removal of secretions, during periods of superimposed chest infection, may be helpful. IPPB may be contra-indicated if cavitation has taken place. Breathing control should be encouraged to overcome breathlessness.

A *tuberculoma* is a cavity with thick walls containing inspissated material which appears radiologically as a rounded opacity. It may be removed surgically since it is sometimes difficult to differentiate tuberculoma from carcinoma.

Tuberculous bronchiectasis may be a complication of either primary or post-primary tuberculosis. Postural drainage may be given, but clapping will be contra-indicated if there is a large cavity or haemoptysis. The physiotherapist should stand behind the patient when he is coughing. Treatment is carried out two or three times daily according to the quantity of sputum.

MISCELLANEOUS PULMONARY DISORDERS

OCCUPATIONAL LUNG DISEASE

Several lung diseases are attributable to the inhalation of dusts, fumes or noxious substances. The most common of these 'occupational' lung diseases are *coal-miners' pneumoconiosis* and *silicosis*.

Fibrotic nodules develop throughout the lungs around the particles of inhaled dust and these progress to large areas of fibrosis. The diseases may be complicated by chronic bronchitis and emphysematous changes. Symptoms include progressive dyspnoea on exertion, accompanied by cough which may be productive of mucoid sputum and recurrent exacerbations of bronchitis.

The most important aspect of management of these diseases is prevention by adequate precautions in industry and regular chest radiography for employees exposed to risk.

The aims of physiotherapy are similar to those for chronic bronchitis and emphysema, assistance with removal of secretions by postural drainage and possibly IPPB (p. 120) and instruction in breathing with economy of effort (p. 47).

DIFFUSE FIBROSING ALVEOLITIS

This condition is characterized by a diffuse inflammatory process in the lung beyond the terminal bronchiole, resulting in thickening and fibrosis of the alveolar walls. This may occur rapidly in the subacute form known as the Hamman–Rich syndrome and it may be fatal within 6 months. More commonly the disease progresses in the chronic form over a few years.

The characteristic symptom is progressive and unremitting dyspnoea. Pulmonary function tests show a restrictive defect with reduction in gas exchange. Radiographs show fine, diffuse mottling.

Steroids may limit the fibrosis and relieve dyspnoea in some patients. Physiotherapy is purely palliative. Instruction in breathing control may give some relief. If superimposed infections occur, IPPB and chest vibrations may assist removal of secretions. Use of the high frequency oscillator may relieve breathlessness and may help to mobilize excess bronchial secretions.

RHEUMATOID DISEASE AND ASSOCIATED CONDITIONS

Many of the diseases allied to rheumatoid disease show respiratory manifestations and those producing symptoms may benefit from physiotherapy.

In *rheumatoid arthritis* there may be pleural effusion and pleural thickening, pulmonary nodules and diffuse interstitial fibrosis. The patient may have radiographic changes, but be asymptomatic or symptoms of dyspnoea and cough may develop. The presence of bronchopulmonary infection may be masked by anti-inflammatory drugs.

In *systemic lupus erythematosus* (SLE) pleurisy with or without an effusion often occurs accompanied by acute pleuritic pain. There may be pneumonic changes either directly due to SLE or secondary to an infection. Radiographic changes show gradual elevation of the diaphragm. This progressive lung 'shrinkage' may be caused by dysfunction of the diaphragm rather than primary pathology of the lung (Gibson *et al.* 1977). Lung function tests indicate a restrictive defect with reduced total lung capacity, vital capacity, lung compliance and often a reduction in diffusing capacity.

Both these conditions are treated with

corticosteroids, but symptomatic treatment by the physiotherapist may be beneficial. Instruction in breathing control is given to relieve dyspnoea at rest and on exertion and thoracic expansion exercises help to maintain mobility of the thoracic cage. In cases of SLE with grossly reduced vital capacity, IPPB may assist movement of the thoracic cage or loosen secretions if they are present. In the event of an infection necessitating more vigorous physiotherapy in rheumatoid arthritis, it is advisable to consider the possibility of steroid-induced osteoporosis.

The same principles of treatment apply to other associated conditions such as systemic sclerosis (generalized scleroderma) and polyarteritis nodosa.

Ankylosing spondylitis is an acquired disease of the spine and sacroiliac joints. During the later stages of the disease the vertebral joints become immobile and the thorax becomes fixed causing a restrictive pulmonary defect.

A patient referred for physiotherapy early in the disease benefits from mobility exercises for the spine and thorax and thoracic expansion exercises to maintain movement of the rib cage. A patient whose thorax has become fixed may require assistance if he develops a bronchopulmonary infection. IPPB, with a relatively high pressure to overcome the resistance of the rib cage, may help clear bronchial secretions.

PULMONARY REACTIONS TO THE ASPERGILLUS

The aspergillus is a common fungus which causes various types of pulmonary disease. The spores of the fungus are present in the atmosphere and are particularly prevalent in Great Britain in the winter months.

In some people the aspergillus causes an immediate allergic response producing an attack of *asthma*. In these cases there is an instant positive reaction to skin testing.

In others a more complex allergic response occurs producing a disease known as *allergic bronchopulmonary aspergillosis*. Skin testing produces an immediate and a delayed response. The symptoms include inflammation and oedema of the bronchi and bronchioli which cause wheezing. Transient pulmonary infiltrates develop associated with pulmonary eosinophilia and often lead to obstruction of the bronchi and collapse of a segment or lobe. Eventually bronchiectasis may develop with fixed airflow obstruction. The sputum may contain bronchial casts, often brown in colour, from which *Aspergillus fumigatus* can be cultured.

Treatment is similar to that for asthma. Postural drainage may take longer than usual if the patient has bronchial casts, but great relief is felt once they are expectorated. IPPB or PCPAP with a bronchodilator preceding postural drainage is useful to relieve bronchospasm and to assist in loosening secretions. Inhalation from an ultrasonic nebulizer, or another type of efficient humidifier, preceding postural drainage often assists expectoration (p. 138).

Aspergillus fumigatus may infect cysts or cavities which have resulted from such diseases as tuberculosis, pulmonary infarction or lung abscess. An *aspergilloma* is a solid ball of fungus (mycetoma) which fills the cavity. Radiography will demonstrate a crescent of air above the opacity which can be shown to alter position with changes of posture.

Some patients have recurrent haemoptysis while others are asymptomatic. Surgery is rarely undertaken because of the risk of spreading the fungal infection. An aspergilloma is often treated medically, but where haemoptyses are severe resection may be necessary.

Occasionally a patient with an aspergilloma becomes sensitive to the aspergillus in the cavity and then develops a cough, wheeze, sputum and other symptoms of allergic bronchopulmonary aspergillosis.

Inhalations of antifungal agents such as natamycin (Pimafucin) or Brilliant Green, are sometimes prescribed in the treatment of aspergilloma or allergic bronchopulmonary aspergillosis.

HUMAN IMMUNODEFICIENCY VIRUS (HIV)—AIDS

Pulmonary infections are commonly associated with AIDS. Immunodeficiency allows pathogens that would normally be fended off to cause opportunistic infections. Examples of these pathogens are Pneumocystis carinii or cytomegalovirus.

AIDS is characterized at first by general non-specific symptoms such as fever, fatigue and weight loss. Respiratory symptoms develop weeks or months later and are usually dyspnoea and non-productive cough. Chest radiographs may show interstitial shadowing and typical changes in lung function are a reduction in vital capacity, total lung capacity and diffusing capacity.

Pulmonary infections are often diagnosed by transbronchial biopsy or bronchoalveolar lavage performed by fibreoptic bronchoscopy, but sometimes the diagnosis can be made from sputum examination. It is often difficult for the patient to produce sputum, but inhalation of hypertonic saline from a nebulizer has been found helpful (Bigby et al. 1986).

If excess bronchial secretions become apparent, physiotherapy to assist clearance of secretions should be given. Physiotherapy may also be required to assist in mobilizing the patient who suffers from severe muscle weakness.

PULMONARY TUMOURS

Carcinoma of the bronchus is the most common tumour of the lung. The majority of these tumours arise centrally in the larger bronchi and are visible through a bronchoscope. A few develop peripherally. Histologically 56% are found to be squamous cell carcinoma, 37% are anaplastic (oat cell carcinoma), 6% adenocarcinoma and 1% alveolar cell carcinoma.

The first symptoms are often a dry cough and pain, but as the growth increases in size it causes progressive bronchial obstruction and production of mucopurulent sputum, leading eventually to collapse of the lung segment. Haemoptysis may result from ulceration of blood vessels and a persistent wheeze becomes apparent due to obstruction of the bronchus. Complications such as unresolved pneumonia, lung abscess or pleural effusion are not uncommon.

Surgery by lobectomy or pneumonectomy is often the treatment of choice (p. 79), but if the growth is too extensive, or too rapidly progressive (anaplastic), or the respiratory reserve is inadequate, other methods are employed.

Chemotherapy and/or radiotherapy may be used to produce a remission in patients unsuitable for resection, or to relieve symptoms such as obstruction of the superior vena cava. If there is infection beyond the bronchial obstruction the patient will start to expectorate purulent sputum once the tumour reduces in size. Physiotherapy, by means of postural drainage, breathing exercises and gentle vibratory shaking can help the removal of secretions. More vigorous technique are contra-indicated in view of possible haemoptysis or the presence of metastases in the spine or ribs.

As a result of radiotherapy, pulmonary fibrosis may develop causing dyspnoea. Instruction in breathing control in the high side-lying resting position and with walking often provides relief.

Physiotherapy may be requested for patients in the terminal stage of the disease to assist with removal of secretions. Postural drainage (or a modified form) with gentle vibrations may be helpful if a patient is distressed and having difficulty in clearing the airways. IPPB is contra-indicated if the tumour is partially obstructing a large bronchus as air trapping may result, but it could be used to assist clearance of bronchial secretions if the tumour is in the peripheral airways. If the patient is unable to cough and expectorate, is alert and in extreme distress, nasotracheal suction may on rare occasions be used, but it is unjustified during the terminal stage if the patient is in a state of coma.

Adenoma and *hamartoma* are benign tumours of the lung treated by surgical removal.

PULMONARY EMBOLISM

A pulmonary embolus most commonly arises from a deep vein thrombosis in the leg or pelvis. A distinction must be drawn between massive pulmonary embolism where more than 50% of the major pulmonary artery branches are obstructed and pulmonary infarct caused by several small emboli.

Massive pulmonary embolism

A large embolus may cause sudden death. If the embolism is not immediately fatal the patient becomes suddenly shocked, dyspnoeic and complains of central chest pain. Pulmonary angiography may be used to confirm the diagnosis. Treatment may be either by intravenous anti-coagulants or emergency embolectomy. Surgery is carried out on cardiopulmonary bypass (p. 106).

Pulmonary infarction

Small emboli cause a pulmonary infarct. Diagnosis is often difficult and this serious respiratory lesion is sometimes overlooked. When the infarct extends to the lung surface, the pleura becomes involved causing acute pleuritic pain and often effusion. Haemoptysis occurs only in about 50% of cases and the source of the embolus is not always clinically detectable. Repeated small emboli may eventually lead to obstruction of the pulmonary vascular bed and cause pulmonary hypertension and right ventricular failure.

Treatment of pulmonary infarction consists of anti-coagulants, oxygen, bed rest and analgesia to relieve the pleuritic pain. The patient is mobilized as soon as the physician consents.

Physiotherapy is primarily prophylactic and all patients at risk are given instruction in active leg exercises and breathing exercises to assist the venous return. Patients are encouraged to carry out foot and leg exercises at frequent intervals until they are ambulant.

If a pulmonary infarct occurs, physiotherapy is discontinued until anti-coagulant therapy is established. Breathing exercises are then given to encourage movement of the affected area since chest movement is limited by the pleuritic pain. Postural drainage may assist expectoration of old blood and clot. Leg exercises are continued until the patient is ambulant.

DISEASES OF THE PLEURAL CAVITY

PLEURAL EFFUSION

Breathing exercises are important following a pleural effusion to maintain mobility of the thoracic cage before adhesions form and the pleura becomes thickened. The types of pleural effusion most commonly seen by the physiotherapist are those found in association with pneumonia, tuberculosis and trauma and those following thoracic surgery. Pleural effusion may also be associated with cardiac failure, nephritis or intrathoracic neoplasms. These conditions do not benefit from physiotherapy.

If there is a large effusion causing dyspnoea, breathing exercises are not usually effective until the fluid has been aspirated. Thoracic expansion exercises are given to all areas of the affected side of the chest, including the apical area where there is often some flattening. Belt exercises (p. 19) may be useful in this condition. If there is gross deformity of the chest wall, the patient is positioned lying on the unaffected side with two or three pillows under the thorax in order to open out the rib cage of the affected side. Breathing exercises are done intermittently while in this position. It may be necessary to lie in the position for 20 to 30 minutes several times a day.

EMPYEMA

Empyema, a collection of pus in the pleural cavity, is now rarely seen. It may be associated with bronchopleural fistula following pulmonary surgery. Empyema may be treated surgically by decortication (p. 95) or rib resection with insertion of a drainage tube or medically. If patients are treated medically by chemotherapy and possibly aspiration, thoracic expansion exercises are part of the general treatment regimen. Empyema results in thickening of the pleura and restriction of lung movement. Early physiotherapy is essential so that maximum re-expansion of lung tissue and minimum permanent restriction result. Breathing exercises are necessary to prevent deformities, as with pleural effusion.

SPONTANEOUS PNEUMOTHORAX

A collection of air in the pleural cavity resulting from some pathological process is known as spontaneous pneumothorax. When the pneumothorax is small the lung often re-expands within a few days. Treatment consists of rest and physiotherapy is usually unnecessary. If the lung fails to re-expand or collapses further, air must be withdrawn from the pleural cavity. An intercostal tube is inserted for a few days and the air in the pleural space withdrawn. Following the insertion of a tube, breathing exercises may be given to assist re-expansion of the lung. Particular attention should be given to expansion of the apical region if there is an apical air pocket. The physiotherapist should ensure that the patient carries out a full range of movements in the shoulder joint on the affected side.

In some cases the spontaneous pneumothorax recurs with consequent chest pain, dyspnoea and interference with day-to-day activities. If any other lung disease is present such as emphysema, a recurrent pneumothorax may result in severe disability. For this reason the pleural cavity is sometimes obliterated medically with talc or irritant oils (pleurodesis) or surgically by pleurectomy or abrasion pleurodesis (p. 95).

CHRONIC HYPERVENTILATION SYNDROME

Chronic hyperventilation syndrome is a clinical disorder with no known organic basis which induces a wide variety of symptoms as a result of episodes of hyperventilation. The symptoms mimic many different organic diseases and the condition is often unrecognized until the patient has been investigated in numerous clinics and has become increasingly anxious.

Hyperventilation causes the respiratory centre to acclimatize to a persistently low level of arterial carbon dioxide. The major effect of a low carbon dioxide level is to cause vasoconstriction and in particular a decrease in cerebral blood flow. This may lead to dizziness, fainting, an inability to concentrate and memory disturbance. Other symptoms that may be present are chest pain (pseudo-angina), palpitations, breathlessness, excessive yawning, swallowing difficulty, indigestion, muscular pains and the feeling of exhaustion unrelated to exertion. The patient may suffer severe anxiety, tension and fear. It is often possible to discover an emotional or physical event that coincides with the start of the disorder.

The patient tends to breathe using mainly the upper chest with increased accessory muscle activity. The breathing pattern is usually irregular in rate and depth with the occurrence of excessive yawning or sighing.

At the start of treatment a simple explanation of the control of respiration and gas exchange will relieve the anxiety of the patient as he realizes that there is a tangible cause for his symptoms. Treatment must not be rushed. It is crucial to take time to talk and listen to the patient and to gain his confidence. While taking a careful history, the precipitating factor may become apparent.

The aim of physiotherapy is to alter the pattern of breathing in order to decrease ventilation and to raise the resting arterial carbon dioxide level. This can be achieved by conscious control of the depth, rate and regularity of respiration (Innocenti 1987). The mass spectrometer or any rapid-response carbon dioxide analyser may be used to give feedback on the level of carbon dioxide in the expired air (Moon 1981).

The patient is first treated in the supine position with the knees bent over pillows to allow relaxation of the abdominal wall. A lower chest breathing pattern is encouraged, with relaxation of the upper chest. Attempts are made to develop a smooth, slow gentle breathing pattern with gradual lengthening of expiration or extension of the pause between expiration and inspiration. Monotonous counting by the physiotherapist and possibly a tape recording for home use may help the patient to develop this 'new' pattern.

The respiratory centre will eventually accept a higher (normal) level of carbon dioxide, but initially during the breathing training the patient may feel a desperate desire for a deep breath. This may be associated with the stretch reflexes in the muscles and joints of the chest wall. Swallowing may relieve this discomfort, but if this is not successful, a technique of breath holding is used. The patient takes a deep breath and then counts for 2 or 3 seconds both at full inspiration and at the end of expiration. This 'breath hold' technique will compensate for the lowering of the carbon dioxide level during the deep breath and can be used whenever the patient has an uncontrollable desire to sigh or yawn. He should try and revert to the controlled breathing pattern after this compensatory breath.

A few patients may be unable to control attacks in times of stress and will need to use an emergency measure. Breathing in and out of a paper bag will relieve the symptoms as re-breathing the expired gas causes the carbon dioxide level to rise.

With patience and practice the new regular breathing pattern will eventually become a natural, subconscious method of breathing.

SPINAL INJURY

The degree of respiratory disability resulting from transection of the spinal cord depends on the level of injury. Lesions above the 4th cervical vertebra (C4) result in paralysis of all the respiratory muscles with the exception of some of the accessory muscles, mainly trapezius and sternomastoid. Patients with these lesions require mechanical ventilation.

With transection of the cervical cord below C4 there is partial or complete function of the diaphragm and scalene muscles, but the intercostal and abdominal muscles are paralysed. Lesions of the upper thoracic spine (T2–T5) result in partial function of the intercostal muscles, but paralysis of the abdominals.

In the tetraplegic patient vital capacity is reduced as a result of weakness of the inspiratory and expiratory muscles and cough is seriously impaired. Expiratory force is generated entirely from the elastic recoil of the lung produced by the previous inspiration.

In a normal subject expiratory force generates a rise in pleural pressure. This produces dynamic compression of the airways, downstream of the equal pressure point (p. 21) and increases the linear velocity of gas flow which assists clearance of bronchial secretions. In the tetraplegic, the paralysed expiratory muscles cannot provide the increased pleural pressure necessary to produce dynamic compression and an increase in linear gas flow.

Normally, dynamic compression of the trachea and major bronchi occurs following an inspiration to high lung volume. The tetraplegic has a reduced lung volume and the equal pressure point cannot reach the largest airways. He may be able to clear the smaller airways, but secretions often lodge in the main airways and trachea (Morgan et al. 1986).

The intercostal muscles normally prevent the intercostal spaces being sucked inwards by the negative intrathoracic pressure produced by contraction of the diaphragm. In the acute stage of cervical injury (below C4) muscle tone is flaccid and paradoxical inward movement of the intercostal spaces may occur, dissipating the energy of the diaphragm. As the intercostal tone increases and the rib cage joints stiffen, paradoxical movement lessens and vital capacity increases.

Two other factors that affect the efficiency of the diaphragm are the curve of the dome of the diaphragm at the start of inspiration and the compliance of the abdominal wall. The diaphragm requires some abdominal resistance to work efficiently. In the supine position the abdominal contents help to increase the dome-shaped configuration, but when the tetraplegic patient is in the sitting position the diaphragm will be flatter than normal if the abdominal muscles have no postural tone. Vital capacity is less in the sitting position than in supine in patients with a floppy abdominal wall. As abdominal tone increases, function of the diaphragm is more efficient. An abdominal binder can be used to provide a similar effect if tone remains diminished. In a few cases, generalized spasm or gross obesity may provide an increased resistance and decrease the efficiency of the diaphragm.

Treatment in the acute stage

Prophylactic physiotherapy is necessary in the acute phase following spinal injury to prevent atelectasis.

The patient's position is changed every 4 hours and breathing exercises are given to encourage thoracic expansion, in the side-lying and supine positions. Clearance of bronchial secretions requires assistance by manual compression of the chest wall, in time with attempts at coughing. The physiotherapist places her hands on the lateral and anterior aspects of the chest wall when the patient is supine.

A large or obese patient may need two physiotherapists, one standing on each side of the bed, to give adequate pressure to produce an effective cough. The hands are placed on the upper and lower ribs, or while using one hand on the upper rib cage the other forearm can give pressure across the lower chest at the level of the diaphragm. The patient takes his maximum breath in and compression of the chest is synchronized as he makes an effort to cough.

If the patient is retaining secretions or has an area of atelectasis, treatment can be assisted by using an intermittent positive pressure breathing machine (IPPB, p. 120) provided that there are no contra-indications (p. 128). The machine is regulated to give an inspiratory volume greater than the patient can achieve voluntarily. The elastic recoil of the lungs is increased at this higher lung volume, expiratory flow improves and assisted coughing is more effective.

When the rib cage stiffens, following spinal injury, the respiratory muscles work at a mechanical disadvantage. IPPB used in the early phase may keep these joints mobile and the muscles better able to work at a mechanical advantage. A patient requiring an endotracheal tube or tracheostomy and mechanical ventilation will probably require manual hyperinflation with chest vibrations to prevent atelectasis (p. 110).

Treatment of the non-acute patient

Assessment of the patient includes observation of the breathing pattern, movement of the chest wall and abdominal muscle tone in the supine and sitting positions. Vital capacity is recorded in these positions and mouth pressure measurements give an estimate of inspiratory and expiratory muscle strength.

Postural drainage, breathing exercises and assisted coughing are used if there are excess bronchial secretions. The patient is taught to give self compression to assist coughing if he has power in his upper limbs. Relatives are instructed in assisted coughing techniques to be used with the patient in the lying and sitting positions.

IPPB may be used to assist clearance of secretions if the patient has a chest infection. With the reduced vital capacity following spinal injury there is a tendency for a reduction in pulmonary and rib cage compliance. If IPPB is used to increase lung volume, the alveoli will retain their elasticity and there is less possibility of microatelectasis and infection. By improving pulmonary and rib cage compliance the work of breathing is lessened.

An alternative to IPPB for assisting clearance of secretions and for improving compliance is glossopharyngeal breathing (p. 142). The patient can use this technique in any position to augment his vital capacity and to produce a much more effective cough. Those patients with poor abdominal tone benefit from wearing an abdominal binder.

Respiratory muscle training may increase strength and endurance of the respiratory muscles and protect against fatigue (Gross *et al.* 1980). Many devices are available with inspiratory and expiratory resistances for endurance or strength training.

7 Surgical conditions

THORACIC SURGERY

This section covers the physiotherapy associated with surgery of the lungs and pleura, but also includes oesophageal and diaphragmatic surgery and correction of chest deformities.

Thoracic surgery is frequently undertaken for patients with bronchial carcinoma, but before the surgeon decides if the case is operable, detailed investigations are performed. In addition to routine history, chest radiograph, electrocardiograph, blood, sputum and lung function tests, more specific investigations are carried out to exclude metastases.

Bronchoscopy is a procedure to examine the airways visually. The instrument is inserted through the mouth or nose and trachea into the bronchi. The flexible fibre-optic bronchoscope, used under local anaesthetic, provides a view of the bronchial tree as far as the sub-segmental orifices. It can be used to obtain a biopsy of lesions for definitive diagnosis. The rigid bronchoscope, which is used less commonly, requires a general anaesthetic and provides vision as far as the segmental bronchi.

Bronchoscopy is most often performed when carcinoma is suspected, but it may also be used to obtain biopsies for diagnostic purposes in patients with diffuse pulmonary disease, to remove mucus plugs or to remove an inhaled foreign body.

Mediastinoscopy or an anterior mediastinotomy may be undertaken under general anaesthetic to determine whether the carcinoma has spread to involve the mediastinal lymph nodes. For mediastinoscopy an instrument is introduced through a small transverse incision above the suprasternal notch. Abnormalities of the superior mediastinum and enlargement of lymph nodes can be detected and biopsies of lymph nodes are taken.

The surgeon may prefer an anterior mediastinotomy to investigate involvement of the mediastinal lymph nodes. A small incision is made in the second intercostal space but no intercostal drainage tubes are inserted. It is advisable for the physiotherapist to encourage pre- and post-operative breathing techniques as described below.

Tomography and computerized tomography (CT) (p. 11) can provide information about the precise location and character of lung lesions. CT scanning is also able to identify invasion of a tumour into the surrounding chest wall and pleura as well as the mediastinum.

Fluoroscopy can be used to show movement of the diaphragm. If one side of the diaphragm is paralysed, it is possible that a tumour has damaged the phrenic nerve.

Angiography is a technique occasionally used to outline the superior vena cava where obstruction of the vessel is suspected.

Ventilation and perfusion scans using

radioisotopes may help detect areas of the lung which are not functioning efficiently. If a scan shows areas that are ventilated, but not perfused, the presence of an embolus is suspected. A section of lung that is both unventilated and unperfused is probably a portion of lung containing a bulla.

Liver, bone and brain scans may be carried out to detect metastases. The surgeon will assess the results of these investigations before deciding whether surgery is indicated. Patients with bronchial carcinoma are considered inoperable if there is mediastinal lymph node involvement, superior vena caval obstruction, recurrent laryngeal nerve palsy or evidence of metastases.

Post-operative lung function cannot be accurately predicted before surgery. Patients whose lung function may be considered critical are those with a vital capacity of less than 50% predicted normal value, or an FEV_1 of less than 1 litre or 50% of FVC, before thoracotomy (Spiro 1986). Some surgeons base their decision to operate on lung function tests while others consider that if a patient can walk up two flights of stairs and is able to talk on arrival, he is able to withstand surgery.

Physiotherapy has an important part to play in the care of patients following thoracic surgery and one of the aids to a quick recovery is adequate pre-operative training. The principles of pre-operative treatment are the same for all patients undergoing thoracic surgery, but vary in detail according to the individual's condition and the operation to be performed. Treatment should start as early as possible.

Before starting pre-operative treatment, the physiotherapist should examine the patient's medical history and chest radiographs and other relevant investigations such as lung function tests. It is important at this stage that the physiotherapist evaluates the patient's normal breathing pattern, thoracic mobility and range of shoulder movement. These observations should be recorded as they will be of value in the post-operative phase.

Following thoracic and abdominal surgery a restrictive pattern of lung function develops and remains for up to 14 days post-operatively. There is a marked reduction in FEV_1 and FVC and a slight decrease in functional residual capacity (FRC). It is this change in FRC which is probably the most important as it causes small airway closure (Craig 1981) impairing gas exchange and leading to hypoxaemia. Prolonged small airway closure will be followed by atelectasis of a lung segment or lung.

Breathing exercises (p. 16), mechanical adjuncts (p. 120 and 129) and the use of positioning which will increase tidal volume and in particular FRC are encouraged, to modify the post-operative changes.

Prophylactic chest physiotherapy has been shown to reduce the frequency of post-operative chest infection in abdominal surgery (Morran *et al.* 1983).

Aims of physiotherapy following thoracic surgery

1 To preserve adequate ventilation.
2 To assist removal of excess secretions to minimize the occurrence of atelectasis and chest infection.
3 To maintain or regain full expansion of the remaining lung tissue.
4 To assist the circulation of the legs and

thereby help prevent post-operative venous thrombosis.

5 To maintain mobility of the shoulders, shoulder girdle, spine and chest.

6 To prevent postural deformity.

7 To restore exercise tolerance.

PRE-OPERATIVE TRAINING

1 Explanation to the patient

During the pre-operative period the physiotherapist should gain the patient's confidence. It should be explained that, to maintain adequate ventilation of the lungs, breathing exercises must be performed. These will inevitably be uncomfortable. Analgesia will be given, but this does not eliminate pain entirely and the patient must understand the importance of clearing secretions in the airways after surgery, in order to prevent post-operative complications.

Reassurance must be given that deep breathing, huffing, coughing and moving around in bed will not harm the stitches, drainage tubes or operation site.

The patient should also realize the importance of starting his exercises as soon as he recovers consciousness after surgery and that physiotherapy is of the greatest importance during the first few post-operative days.

2 Removal of secretions

The lungs should be as clear as possible before surgery and any excess secretions should be removed by appropriate postural drainage. If bronchiectasis is present, intensive physiotherapy will probably be necessary.

Cigarette smoking causes bronchoconstriction and excess secretions. The patient should be encouraged to stop smoking.

Bronchitis often co-exists with bronchial carcinoma and some patients may be too dyspnoeic to tolerate the postural drainage positions for the lung bases. Modified positions should be used (p. 29).

3 Breathing control (p. 15)

Breathing control using the lower chest helps the patient to return to the normal pattern of breathing. The upper chest and shoulder girdle must be relaxed. Breathing control should be encouraged between the more active breathing exercises and may assist the loosening of secretions in the lower zones of the lungs.

4 Breathing exercises

Thoracic expansion exercises (p. 17) mobilize bronchial secretions, assist re-expansion of remaining lung tissue and help to prevent the formation of air pockets. A lateral thoracotomy is used for the majority of operations included in this section. With the exception of pneumonectomy, the patient will be required to emphasize lower lateral thoracic expansion for the side of the incision as movement of this side will be inhibited by pain. Unilateral expansion of the unaffected side should also be practised. Holding full inspiration for 3 seconds helps to increase aeration of the alveoli (Ward et al. 1966). This should be repeated four times before returning to breathing control. Longer periods of thoracic expansion exercises may lead to hyperventilation, but the cycle can be repeated several times.

Most pulmonary surgery is performed for bronchial carcinoma. The surgeon

81

may not be able to predict the extent of an operation until the chest has been opened. Lobectomy may be possible or pneumonectomy may be necessary. Occasionally the growth is so extensive that it is inoperable, but this finding is rare with the careful selection procedure for surgery. Pre-operatively the patient practises unilateral thoracic expansion for each side of the chest. The emphasis post-operatively will depend on the surgical procedure. It is the surgeon, not the physiotherapist, who should tell the patient the details of the operation.

5 The forced expiration technique and coughing

Huffing combined with breathing control helps to loosen and clear bronchial secretions.

Many patients find huffing more comfortable than coughing. Huffing at high lung volume can be a substitute for much coughing. Huffing from mid lung volume to low lung volume is used to clear progressively deeper parts of the airways.

The patient must be aware of the difference between an effective huff or cough and a noise created in the throat. The physiotherapist should attune herself to the various sounds that patients make, so that she is not misled by a dry coughing noise when secretions might be heard and shifted if the huff or cough was deeper and more effective.

The physiotherapist should show the patient how she will support the chest firmly below the incision for a lateral thoracotomy with counter-pressure given anteriorly (fig. 71). At the same time the patient can press the hand of the unaffected side against the painful area of the side of his chest.

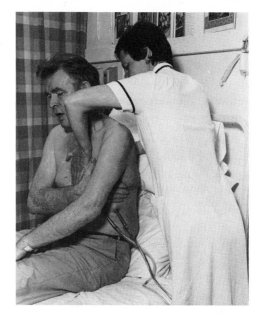

Fig. 71. *Lateral thoracotomy supported by physiotherapist.*

An alternative method of support that the physiotherapist can use if manual pressure is not adequate, is to place a folded towel around the chest wall just above the site of the intercostal drains.

The patient is also instructed in supporting his chest when needing to huff and cough without an assistant. He uses his hand and arm to give pressure by placing the arm of the unaffected side across the front of the chest, the hand giving pressure just below the incision and the other elbow giving pressure inwards to the chest wall (fig. 72).

The breathing techniques should be practised by the patient during the pre-operative period.

6 Foot and leg exercises

All patients should be taught simple foot and ankle exercises and knee flexion and

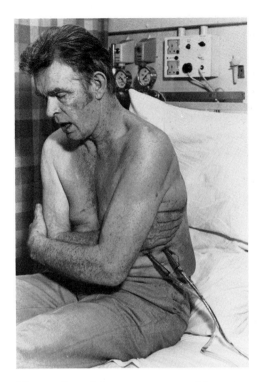

Fig. 72. *Lateral thoracotomy supported by patient during a huff.*

The tendency to side-flex the trunk towards the incision and to lower the affected shoulder should be pointed out to the patient. The importance of correcting this tendency and preventing any permanent defect should be explained (fig. 73).

8 Arm and shoulder girdle movements

Any restriction in shoulder joint movement should be recorded pre-operatively. The prevention of loss of joint range and mobility by early post-operative shoulder girdle and arm exercises should be explained to the patient. Simple shoulder girdle and arm exercises should be practised briefly. Resisted movement with proprioceptive neuromuscular facilitation techniques are helpful in gaining full range with minimal pain. It is of value to practise a few movements with this technique pre-operatively.

9 Moving in bed

It is helpful to show the patient how to move himself up the bed taking his weight

extension to assist the circulation and help prevent post-operative venous thrombosis. It should be emphasized that unless the patient is ambulant these exercises should be practised during every waking hour.

7 Posture

The habitual standing posture of the patient should be noted in order that a comparison can be made with posture during the post-operative period.

Patients are ambulant soon after surgery and problems of postural deformity rarely arise, but children and young adults sometimes find difficulty in maintaining good posture after lateral thoracotomy.

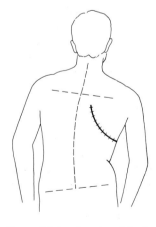

Fig. 73. *Postural deformity after right thoracotomy.*

83

on his unaffected arm so that he can be mobile without pulling on his drainage tubes and causing pain.

POST-OPERATIVE TREATMENT

Before starting treatment, the physiotherapist should read the operation notes to find the details of the procedure performed.

Before each treatment the patient should be observed and his record charts studied:

1 Colour, cyanosis.
2 Respiratory rate.
3 Temperature and pulse.
4 Blood pressure.
5 Observe the number and site of the pleural drainage tubes and whether they are connected to suction. Note the amount of drainage and whether there is bubbling or swing in the bottles.
6 Arterial blood gas results, if available.
7 Sputum expectorated: colour and quantity.
8 Chest radiograph.
9 Analgesia: note if the patient had cryoanalgesia during surgery and the method of giving post-operative analgesia. Is it a continuous intravenous infusion which may need to be increased before physiotherapy or is he having intermittent injections? Note the time the last dose was given.
10 It is important to listen to the breath sounds before and after treatment.

Post-operative treatment should start after return to the ward, when the patient is sufficiently conscious and cooperative. He should be encouraged to do his breathing exercises and then, while firmly supported, be helped to huff and cough. Often he will cough better at this stage than on the following day as there may be residual analgesia and sedation from the anaesthetic.

Treatment is probably necessary four times during the day, but the patient is also encouraged to practise his breathing techniques and leg exercises for a few minutes in every hour that he is awake. He should be sitting up in bed with his back well supported by pillows so that lower chest movements are not inhibited.

After about 24 hours the patient will usually be allowed to sit out of bed for periods. The exercises can be carried out satisfactorily in this position.

Treatment should include:

1 Breathing control and breathing exercises

(a) Breathing control.
(b) Unilateral lower thoracic expansion for each side of the chest with emphasis on the operation side (except after pneumonectomy). A breath hold of 3 seconds at full inspiration is encouraged.
(c) Apical expansion if appropriate. If there is an apical intercostal drainage tube and/or upper lobe lung tissue has been removed, apical expansion exercises may be helpful. This exercise helps to prevent the formation of an apical airpocket and assists re-expansion of the remaining lung tissue.

2 The forced expiration technique and coughing

Effective huffing and coughing, as taught pre-operatively (p. 82), must be encouraged with the chest firmly supported. The patient often finds it easier while sitting forwards in bed away from the pillows. When helping to sit the patient forward, support should be given behind the neck to avoid pulling on the painful arm.

If bronchospasm is present, a bronchodilator may be necessary before treatment.

3 Shoulder movements

Shoulder movements should be started the morning after the operation. Resistance given with proprioceptive neuromuscular facilitation techniques is helpful in achieving a good range of movement with minimal pain.

4 Foot and leg exercises

The exercises taught pre-operatively should be practised and the patient should be reminded to do each exercise 5–10 times every hour that he is awake.

5 Postural drainage

If the chest radiograph is satisfactory, there are no sounds of bronchial breathing on auscultation and the patient is able to breathe deeply and to huff and cough effectively, there is probably no need to put him through the unnecessary discomfort of postural drainage.

If the patient is having difficulty clearing bronchial secretions, postural drainage will probably be necessary. Some surgeons leave the decision to the physiotherapist, others prefer to be consulted first.

The drainage position helpful at this stage (except for pneumonectomy, p. 92) is with the patient positioned in sidelying, turned on to his unaffected side, supported by pillows and the foot of the bed raised. The degree to which the bed is tipped depends on the condition of the patient. The shoulder should not rest on the head pillows and the arm on the operated side should be supported by a pillow. Another pillow should be placed behind the back under the drainage tubes to give further support (fig. 74).

The physiotherapist should stand behind the patient during the postural drainage treatment to give effective support during huffing and coughing, effective resistance during the thoracic expansion exercises and to observe the drainage tubes and bottles throughout the treatment.

A patient with bronchiectasis should have postural drainage on the first or second post-operative day.

OTHER FACTORS TO BE CONSIDERED

Analgesia

Adequate analgesia is essential if physiotherapy is to be effective. During surgery

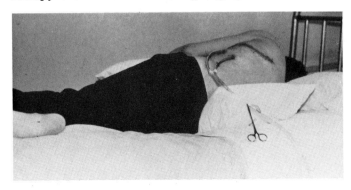

Fig. 74. *Pillows supporting the drainage tubes.*

cryoanalgesia is sometimes used, but additional intravenous or intramuscular analgesics are required during the first 24–36 hours post-operatively. If the patient is on a continuous analgesic by intravenous infusion it is often necessary to increase the rate of infusion to a higher prescribed dose for a few minutes before physiotherapy and until the end of treatment. These drugs may lower the blood pressure and the physiotherapist must make sure that the patient's blood pressure is stable before increasing the dosage.

After 24–36 hours post-operatively analgesia will be changed to oral drugs. Some surgeons prescribe an analgesic and an anti-inflammatory drug. This combination often gives greater pain relief to the patient than the analgesic alone. If adequate analgesia is not attained and the patient is not due for systemic drugs, Entonox by inhalation may assist physiotherapy.

Humidification

High humidity, by means of inhalation before physiotherapy, may help in loosening tenacious secretions (p. 139). A simple steam inhalation may be effective provided the patient inspires deeply, but precautions must be taken to avoid spilling the hot water.

The patient may be dehydrated at this early stage and sometimes a drink helps with coughing and expectoration.

Drainage tubes

After most operations with lateral thoracotomy incisions there will be at least two drainage tubes from the pleural cavity to underwater seal drainage bottles. The basal tube drains mostly fluid and the apical tube allows air leaking from lung tissue into the pleural space to escape, keeping the lung expanded. The basal tube is usually removed within 24–48 hours of surgery. The apical drain (or drains) remains until there is no air leak. This is noted by any air bubbling through the drainage bottles during coughing. If it is removed too early, a pneumothorax results and another tube may have to be inserted.

Each tube is connected via an air-tight bung to a bottle partly filled with sterile water so that air cannot enter the pleura. This is known as an underwater seal. The bottle has an open tube to allow displacement of air. As air comes out of the pleural cavity it bubbles through the water and out of the bottle (fig. 75).

To help keep the remaining lung expanded, the exit tube is usually connected to a suction pump so that a negative pressure is maintained in the bottle. The negative pressure should be increased if a large air leak is present. When the drainage tube is connected to suction there should be no swing of the fluid in the tube in the drainage bottle.

If no suction pump is used, there is still a slight negative pressure in the pleural space which sucks the water a little way up the tube. The fluid level should swing freely with the patient's breathing rising on inspiration and falling on expiration. If there is no swing of the fluid level with quiet breathing, either the lung is fully expanded or the tube has become blocked. A chest radiograph will differentiate between the two.

The drainage tubes from the patient to the bottles should be long enough to allow free movement both in bed and out of bed into a chair. The patient should be encouraged to move about as much as

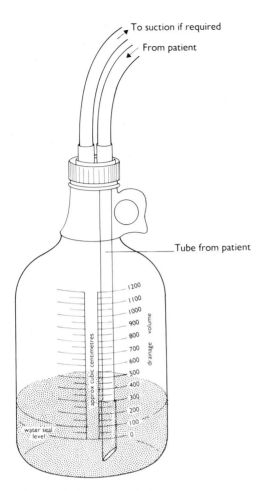

To suction if required

From patient

Tube from patient

1200
1100
1000
900
800
700
600
500
400
300
200
100
0

approx cubic centimetres

drainage volume

water seal level

Fig. 75. *Underwater seal drainage.*

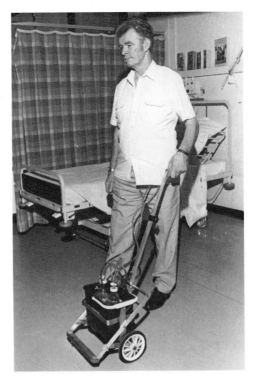

Fig. 76. *Mobility with intercostal drainage tubes.*

possible. If the drainage tubes are not connected to a suction pump, the patient can be encouraged to walk around pushing a small trolley which holds the drainage bottles (fig. 76), or he can carry them at a level lower than the drainage site in his chest.

The tubes should not be clamped during physiotherapy and care must be taken not to pull and disconnect them during movement or to allow them to become kinked. The tubes should be clamped if it

is necessary to move the drainage bottles above the level of the patient, for example during transit or when transferring the bottles to the other side of the bed. If a large air leak is present the clamp should be released as quickly as possible.

If by accident a tube should become disconnected, the part connected to the patient should be clamped and reconnected to the drainage bottles immediately. The clamp should then be removed and the fluid level checked. If there is any cause for concern the medical staff should be informed. Following removal of the pleural drains a radiograph is taken to exclude a pneumothorax. It is preferable to await the result of the radiograph before the next physiotherapy session.

NB: This system of drainage tubes does not apply to pneumonectomy cases (p. 93).

Intermittent positive pressure breathing (IPPB) or periodic continuous positive airway pressure (PCPAP)

If the patient retains secretions and is unable to cough effectively despite all methods described above, it may be necessary to combine treatment with IPPB or PCPAP to assist lung expansion and mobilization of secretions (pp. 126 & 129). Pressure with IPPB must be kept low (below 14 cm H_2O) to prevent an increase in air leak. These adjuncts must only be used with the agreement of the surgeon concerned.

Nasopharyngeal suction

If a patient is still unable to cough effectively and has sputum retention, nasopharyngeal suction will be required to stimulate coughing and assist in removal of secretions (p. 140).

It must be emphasized that this is rarely necessary and is unpleasant for the patient. A frail patient who is likely to require nasopharyngeal suction over a period of more than 24 hours may be more comfortable with a minitracheotomy (p. 141).

THIRD DAY AFTER OPERATION

The number of treatments is reduced according to the patient's condition, but the patient must continue to practise his exercises several times a day.

Treatment includes:

1 *Breathing techniques* as above. These can be carried out sitting in a chair. As soon as unilateral expansion of the affected side is achieved, bilateral expansion (p. 19) can be added (pneumonectomy excepted).

2 *Effective huffing and coughing.*

3 *Shoulder girdle and shoulder movements.* Exercises should include active movements through as full a range as possible. When the drainage tubes have been removed full range of movement should be achieved.

4 *Foot and leg exercises* are continued until the patient is walking around several times a day. If the patient requires intercostal drainage tubes after the second post-operative day, knee-bending exercises from the standing position are introduced. Young patients requiring intercostal suction for several days, for example following pleurectomy (p. 95), benefit from exercising up and down two steps for 2 minutes three or four times daily until the drainage tubes are removed. Portable steps are useful for this purpose. This exercise assists general fitness and also aids re-expansion of lung tissue.

5 *Postural drainage if necessary.* Moderately vigorous activity, for example climbing stairs (if the drainage tubes have been removed) or walking immediately prior to postural drainage, is helpful in loosening secretions by stimulating deeper breathing. Postural drainage is discontinued when the radiograph shows satisfactory re-expansion and sputum has decreased.

6 *Posture* is corrected if necessary.

7 *Simple trunk mobility exercises* can be included.

8 *Walking and increasing activity* should be encouraged.

Exercises as for the third day should be continued, but the number of sessions with the physiotherapist should be reduced as soon as possible. Walking upstairs should be introduced when the drainage tubes have been removed. Breathing control with walking should be taught when necessary.

BEFORE DISCHARGE

Thoracic expansion (except following pneumonectomy), shoulder mobility and posture should have returned to normal. Exercise tolerance should be restored and after operations such as decortication of the lung and plication of bullae it may be markedly improved.

The patient should continue breathing exercises for 3–4 weeks following the operation, although he will probably be discharged after 8–10 days. These should consist of thoracic expansion exercises to the appropriate areas to help in restoring maximum respiratory function and to prevent chest deformity.

If pain persists following thoracotomy, transcutaneous nerve stimulation (TNS) and/or thoracic mobilizations may be helpful.

COMPLICATIONS OF THORACIC SURGERY

1 Sputum retention

This is the most common complication of pulmonary surgery. If secretions are not removed, atelectasis of varying sized areas of lung tissue and/or chest infection may follow. Physiotherapy is aimed at preventing these complications, but if they should occur intensive physiotherapy is essential.

2 Persistent pneumothorax

If an air leak persists for more than 48 hours following surgery, an alveolar or bronchiolar leak should be suspected. The leak occurs from alveoli or bronchioli adjacent to the area of lung resected. A pneumothorax may be visible radiologically. Alveolar leaks heal quickly once the raw surface of lung comes against the chest wall, but bronchiolar leaks persist longer and may require resuturing.

It may be necessary to insert another tube if the drainage tube has already been removed and air is accumulating in the pleural cavity. If no drainage tube is in place and the pneumothorax is increasing in size, a tension pneumothorax may develop and physiotherapy should be discontinued until an intercostal tube has been reinserted.

If a pneumothorax is allowed to remain for a prolonged period, it is a potential source of infection and may result in an empyema. If a small apical pneumothorax is present (with or without a drainage tube in place), expansion exercises should be given, particularly over the apical area and the patient should be instructed to hold full inspiration slightly longer than usual. In the case of a large apical pneumothorax (with a drainage tube in place) showing no signs of reduction in size, the patient should be positioned on his unaffected side with the foot of the bed raised to a height of about 45 cm (18 in). In this position, expansion exercises for the apical area should be practised and may assist in reducing the air space. If a basal air pocket persists, it is sometimes helpful to lie the patient on his affected side for short periods throughout the day. This may release air from a loculated air pocket. Before doing this, adequate analgesia must be given and care must be taken not to occlude or kink the drainage tubes.

3 Surgical emphysema

If air pressure builds up in the pleural space as a result of a communication between the lungs and pleura, air may track into the tissue layers producing subcutaneous or surgical emphysema. A crackling sensation is apparent when the area is palpated. It usually starts around the site of a drainage tube or suture line and may spread into adjacent tissues causing swelling of the chest wall and neck, extending in severe cases to the face and eyelids.

This condition usually subsides with correct tube management, but the physiotherapist must take care not to aggravate the condition. During coughing the glottis is closed, the intrathoracic pressure raised and therefore more air is likely to escape into the tissues. Energetic coughing must be avoided if this is increasing the surgical emphysema. The loosening and removal of bronchial secretions that are present must be assisted by breathing exercises and huffing, without coughing.

4 Bronchopleural fistula

A bronchopleural fistula is a communication between the bronchus and pleural cavity. This is a hazardous complication and occasionally occurs as a result of infection and disruption of the bronchial stump a week or 10 days after pneumonectomy, or more rarely after lobectomy.

The signs of a fistula are a sharp rise in pulse rate, swinging temperature, irritating cough and increase in sputum which may be blood stained. This may be followed by the sudden expectoration of large amounts of brown foul smelling fluid and eventually pus from the infected space.

Treatment consists of aspiration of infected fluid or the insertion of a drainage tube, instillation of antibiotics and postural drainage. Care must be taken to avoid infecting the remaining lung tissue. Resuturing of the bronchial stump may be necessary if healing does not occur. With bronchopleural fistula after pneumonectomy there is a serious risk of flooding the remaining lung with infected pleural fluid. It is essential that the physiotherapist keeps the remaining lung clear and great care must be taken when positioning the patient to prevent any 'spill over' of fluid. The patient should always turn with the affected side at a lower level than the unaffected side.

Following lobectomy it may be safe to drain the remaining segments of the affected lung in the orthodox postural drainage positions, when the fluid has been drained by insertion of an intercostal tube. The affected side should be drained first and the unaffected side drained afterwards in case there has been any 'spill over'.

5 Pleural effusion

A blood stained effusion always collects after resection and the purpose of the basal tube is to drain this fluid. Aspiration may be necessary if fluid reaccumulates after removal of the drainage tube. If excess fluid is allowed to remain, fibrin will be deposited on the visceral pleura causing thickening and restriction of movement. Thoracic expansion exercises should be given to the affected area.

6 Haemothorax

In rare cases haemorrhage into the pleural cavity may occur. This is known as haemothorax. Re-operation may be necessary to seal off bleeding points and remove blood clot from the pleural cavity. Once bleeding has been controlled, breathing exercises should be given to avoid restriction of chest movement due to pleural thickening.

INDIVIDUAL SURGICAL CONDITIONS

Lobectomy

Resection of one or more lobes of a lung.

The pre- and post-operative treatment has been described (p. 80).

If the lobectomy is for bronchiectasis, postural drainage is an essential part of the treatment both before and after surgery.

After lobectomy there will be some displacement of the bronchi as the remaining lung expands to fill the space. Postural drainage positions must be adjusted to find the optimal position for each individual patient.

A simple lobectomy may be performed for bronchial carcinoma, but if the neoplasm has spread into the main bronchus the surgeon may perform a *lobectomy by sleeve resection*. This technique has been devised in order to clear as much tissue as possible into which the neoplasm may have spread, whilst preserving maximum lung function. An end-to-end anastomosis of the main bronchus with the lower lobe bronchus is performed after resecting the affected portion (fig. 77). The patient is more likely to have difficulty in clearing the sputum after this type of operation as the anastomosis may be oedematous and partially occlude the airway. There may be some bleeding into the lower lobe causing thick blood stained secretions. The principles and means of treatment are the same as for a simple lobectomy.

If a bronchial neoplasm has invaded the chest wall, it may be necessary for the surgeon to perform a *lobectomy with partial resection of the chest wall*. In these cases paradoxical chest movement may occur. This is an indrawing of the resected area of chest wall during inspiration with ballooning of the area on expiration. Breathing exercises become difficult and ineffective in these circumstances and a firm 'paradox pad' should be applied to the area to correct this movement. The pad should be made of cotton wool or similar material and be strapped firmly into position.

Severe pain is experienced when a section of the chest wall is resected and analgesia must be given before physiotherapy.

The surgeon may find on opening the thorax that the neoplasm has invaded vital

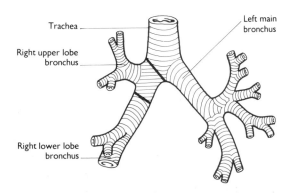

Fig. 77. *Lobectomy by sleeve resection.*

organs or is so extensive as to make lobectomy or pneumonectomy impossible. Pre-operative investigations and careful patient selection make this a rare occurrence, but in this case the thorax is closed leaving one tube in the pleural space to drain post-operative exudate.

Post-operative physiotherapy is the same as for lobectomy. Clearance of secretions may be made difficult if the tumour causes distortion and obstruction of the airways. A few patients with inoperable carcinoma deteriorate rapidly and the physiotherapist should not persist with treatment if this does not relieve the patient's symptoms.

Segmental resection

Removal of a segment of the lung.

A segmental resection may be performed to remove diseased areas of tuberculous lung tissue, non-malignant tumours or cysts.

The pre- and post-operative physiotherapy is as in the general description (p. 80). Although only a small area of lung tissue is removed, the adjoining lung may be affected by surgical trauma during the operation causing more secretions to form. There may be a larger air leak and more exudate draining from the pleural cavity after this operation than after a simple lobectomy. It is common to have blood stained sputum for at least a week after surgery.

Wedge resection

A very small area of lung is removed in order to resect small, non-malignant tumours or cysts such as hamartoma or small hydatid cysts. There is usually no problem with air leak or excessive exudate, but patients are likely to have a moderate amount of sputum.

Pneumonectomy

Total excision of one lung.

Pneumonectomy is most commonly carried out for bronchial carcinoma, but may be necessary for other conditions, for example old tuberculosis with a chronic respiratory infection.

If a patient is definitely scheduled for a pneumonectomy, the physiotherapist can be precise in pre-operative instructions, but if pneumonectomy is only one possibility for a patient with carcinoma undergoing surgery, instructions are less precise.

PRE-OPERATIVE TRAINING

This should include:
1 Explanation of physiotherapy.
2 Removal of excess secretions.
3 Breathing control and breathing exercises:
  (a) breathing control
  (b) lower thoracic expansion for the unaffected side.
4 The forced expiration technique.
5 Effective coughing.
6 Foot and leg exercises.
7 Posture.
8 Arm and shoulder girdle movements.

POST-OPERATIVE TREATMENT

The treatment is essentially the same as that previously described (p. 80) but the following points should be noted:
1 Unilateral lower thoracic expansion

exercises for the remaining lung are emphasized following surgery. Bilateral exercises may be started after 4–5 days to prevent future flattening and rigidity of the chest wall. Equal movement should not be expected.

2 Some patients find difficulty in coughing and tend to strain. It is important to avoid straining during coughing owing to the risk of breakdown of the bronchial suture line and resultant bronchopleural fistula. Patients should therefore loosen the secretions by correct breathing exercises and huffing.

Deviation of the trachea may cause mechanical difficulty with coughing. This is often most marked during the first 24–36 hours following pneumonectomy until the fluid level has begun to stabilize.

3 If the patient cannot clear his secretions in the sitting position he should lie as far over on to the operated side as possible, supported by pillows.

4 If nasopharyngeal suction is required to assist clearance of secretions, great care must be taken when inserting the catheter to avoid contact with the suture line, particularly with a right pneumonectomy. A nasopharyngeal airway, inserted by an anaesthetist, may allow easier access to secretions, but a minitracheotomy (p. 141) is occasionally required if the problem is likely to persist for more than 24–48 hours. The lower end of the minitracheotomy tube must be carefully positioned above the carina.

5 Patients used to be instructed not to lie on the unaffected side of the chest for at least 10 days following pneumonectomy. This allowed time for fibrin to form in the pneumonectomy space and the danger of bronchopleural fistula to have passed. Many surgeons today allow their patients to lie on the unaffected side as soon as the position is comfortable. Bronchopleural fistula is a rare occurrence.

6 The patient usually sits in a chair within 24 hours of the operation and walks within 2 or 3 days. If the postoperative progress is satisfactory, walking upstairs can be started within 1 week, but this depends on the condition of each individual patient. Controlled breathing with walking, on the level and up stairs, should be taught if the patient is dyspnoeic on exertion.

DRAINAGE TUBE

Some surgeons leave a drainage tube in the pleural cavity connected to an underwater seal, for approximately 24 hours. This tube remains clamped and is only released for approximately 1 minute every hour according to instructions. Suction is never applied.

The function of this tube is to control the amount of fluid remaining in the pneumonectomy space and thereby prevent mediastinal shift. If there is too much fluid in the space, there is a shift of the mediastinum towards the remaining lung causing pressure on and partial collapse of the lung. The patient becomes breathless and may develop cardiac arrhythmias due to disturbance of the heart and great vessels in the mediastinum.

If there is too little fluid in the space, the mediastinum shifts away from the remaining lung and again arrhythmias may occur. There will also be overinflation of the remaining lung.

Deviation of the trachea indicates mediastinal shift which can be confirmed radiographically. In order to correct this, it may be necessary for the surgeon to adjust the pressures in the hemithorax. Air can be withdrawn or instilled. Some surgeons like to adjust the fluid level in the hemithorax by routine aspiration so that it is below the level of the bronchial stump, until the danger of bronchopleural fistula has passed.

COMPLICATIONS FOLLOWING PNEUMONECTOMY

1 *Injury to recurrent laryngeal nerve*

During radical pneumonectomy the left recurrent laryngeal nerve is sometimes damaged or may even have to be resected. This results in inability to close the vocal cords and therefore partial loss of effective coughing power. The patient may be able to clear his secretions adequately by breathing exercises and huffing, but the addition of IPPB is often helpful if the surgeon gives permission. Pressure must be kept low, that is no higher than 10 cm H_2O. PCPAP may be a useful alternative.

2 *Phrenic nerve paralysis*

If a tumour involves the phrenic nerve, it may be necessary to resect it causing paralysis of the diaphragm on the affected side. The patient will have an ineffective cough due to the paradoxical movement of the diaphragm. IPPB is helpful in these cases to aerate the lung more effectively and mobilize secretions.

3 *Bronchopleural fistula* (p. 90)

Insertion of radioactive gold grains

When a tumour has been found to be inoperable by resection, the surgeon may implant radioactive gold grains to reduce the size of the growth. This treatment is used in some cases as an alternative to radiotherapy. It may be done either through a thoracotomy or via a bronchoscope.

With a thoracotomy the pre- and post-operative physiotherapy is the same as that for lobectomy.

Post-operatively there is a limit to the time the physiotherapist should stay in the patient's room due to the radioactivity. She must carefully divide her time to allow a few short treatments in the day, or ideally share the treatments with another physiotherapist. The maximum time allowed will increase each day. A monitoring badge should be worn.

The chest radiographs may show gross shadowing due to the radioactivity. Two or 3 days after surgery sputum may increase and contain necrotic material.

If gold grains are introduced via a bronchoscope, coughing should not be encouraged for the first 48 hours.

Plication of emphysematous bullae

If large emphysematous bullae are occupying space in the thoracic cavity, the surgeon may perform a thoracotomy to tie off these bullae to allow the normal lung tissue to expand into the area previously occupied by the cysts. Lung function will be improved as a result.

Instruction in breathing control with relaxation of the upper chest is important. The patients undergoing this type of surgery usually have severe respiratory disability and may experience distress and difficulty in expectoration during the first few post-operative days. They will probably require intensive physiotherapy. Apical breathing is unnecessary as the emphysematous patient will already be over-inflating the upper chest. Walking with controlled breathing on the level and going upstairs should be taught.

Monaldi's procedure is an alternative operation which may be used for emphysematous patients with very poor lung function. It is a less traumatic operation than thoracotomy for plication of bullae. A small incision is made and a Foley catheter is inserted into the bulla for approximately 8 days during which time the bulla collapses and the previously compressed lung tissue fills the space in the thorax.

Pleurectomy

A pleurectomy may be performed if a patient suffers from recurrent pneumothoraces. A small thoracotomy incision is made and the parietal pleura is stripped off the lateral chest wall. As the lung re-expands adhesions form between the chest wall and visceral pleura preventing recurrence of pneumothorax. Blebs or bullae may be oversewn at the same time.

The treatment previously described for thoracotomy is suitable, emphasizing thoracic expansion exercises for the affected side. If a drainage tube is in place pre-operatively for the spontaneous pneumothorax, huffing and coughing can be taught. If there is a partial pneumothorax and no tube in place, huffing and coughing should be demonstrated only. Vigorous coughing could cause an increase in the size of the pneumothorax.

There may not be excess secretions post-operatively when the operation has been performed for idiopathic spontaneous pneumothorax, as there is usually no underlying lung disease. Emphasis must be on thoracic expansion exercises.

If the operation has been performed on a patient with cystic fibrosis, where spontaneous pneumothorax can be a complication, there will be a problem with tenacious secretions. Postural drainage must be started as soon as the patient regains consciousness and will be necessary at least four times a day. Extra humidity may assist expectoration (p. 137).

Abrasion pleurodesis

Abrasion pleurodesis is an alternative surgical procedure for spontaneous pneumothorax. It is performed through a small lateral thoracotomy incision, or sometimes for cosmetic reasons a small vertical mid-axillary incision is used. The pleural surface is rubbed with an abrasive material to produce an inflammatory reaction and subsequent adhesions.

Post-operatively there are one or two drainage tubes in place. Physiotherapy is similar to that for pleurectomy.

Decortication of the lung

If the pleura has become thickened and fibrosed following empyema (tuberculous or non-tuberculous) or haemothorax, the surgeon may perform a thoracotomy and strip off the thickened layers of pleura. If simpler measures have failed to eliminate an empyema cavity, this operation may consist of complete pleurectomy with excision of the empyema cavity. The lung is then free to fill the space formerly occupied by the empyema.

Physiotherapy for thoracotomy applies. Pre-operatively, movement of the chest over the affected area may be very limited and there may be a dramatic improvement after decortication. Rapid expansion of the lung is essential and this is achieved by applying strong suction to the drainage tubes and breathing exercises. Lower thoracic and apical expansion exercises must be emphasized and belt exercises may be necessary to encourage expansion in the later stages of treatment (p. 19).

In patients with extensive tuberculous scarring, the lung may fail to fill the hemithorax completely at the end of the operation. The surgeon may at a later date have to consider thoracoplasty to obliterate the air space.

Lung biopsy

A biopsy of lung tissue is sometimes taken for diagnostic purposes. When it is performed by a percutaneous needle method or by the trans-bronchial method through a fibre-optic bronchoscope, physiotherapy should not be given immediately after the biopsy. A radiograph should be taken to exclude pneumothorax.

Where open lung biopsy is carried out through a thoracotomy physiotherapy, appropriate to the post-operative management of a thoracotomy, is indicated. Although the incision is limited the procedure is often required in patients with a fibrotic lung condition to make a specific diagnosis. Lung function is usually compromised and careful post-operative assessment and treatment is required.

Thoracoplasty

This operation is now rarely required because of advances in the treatment of tuberculosis. It was used formerly as a means of producing permanent collapse of diseased lung tissue to allow healing to take place. It may be used occasionally to obliterate a space in the thoracic cavity, for example in chronic empyema or following resection of lung tissue.

During surgery several ribs are resected subperiosteally. For extensive thoracoplasty which was carried out in two stages, up to 8 ribs including the 1st were resected. When the operation is performed to obliterate a space, the 1st rib is not usually removed and the neck remains more stable because the scalene muscles retain their insertion.

An unsightly scoliosis will occur if correct physiotherapy is not given. It is important that the patient is aware of the deformity likely to occur, and be able to correct it.

PRE-OPERATIVE TRAINING

1 *Breathing control and breathing exercises*

Breathing control, unilateral lower thoracic expansion for each side, the forced expiration technique and coughing should be taught. The patient should be shown how to support the apical area of his chest when he huffs or coughs.

2 *Postural correction in front of a mirror*

The patient will tend to develop a scoliosis with the concavity in the cervical spine and the convexity in the thoracic spine on the side of the operation (fig. 78). He must be taught how to correct these tendencies by means of lateral movement of the neck towards the side of the thoracoplasty, depression of the shoulder girdle on the operation side and correct alignment of the shoulders and pelvis.

3 *Shoulder girdle and arm movements*

Retraction of the scapulae should be taught and full-range arm movements on the side of the thoracoplasty.

Day of operation

Treatment is started as soon as the patient has recovered consciousness and consists of assisted huffing and coughing with firm support over the apical region of the chest wall, breathing control and lower thoracic expansion for each side of the chest. If there is paradoxical movement of the chest wall, a firm pad should be applied below the clavicle extending down into the axilla. The pad should be re-applied regularly by firm bandaging until the paradox has disappeared. Adequate analgesia must be given before physiotherapy.

First day

1 The pillows should be arranged comfortably.
2 Posture should be corrected, but without a mirror at this stage as it may be demoralizing for the patient.
3 Breathing control.
4 Unilateral lower thoracic expansion.
5 Assisted huffing and coughing with firm support below the clavicle to prevent paradox.
6 Active assisted arm movements. These are often more easily performed with a flexed elbow.
7 Depression of the shoulder girdle on the thoracoplasty side.
8 Neck lateral lean towards the thoracoplasty side and it may be helpful to give resistance below the mastoid process.

Second day

1 As above, but if the patient is looking better a mirror may be used.

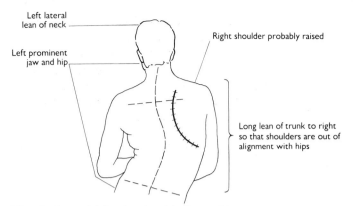

Fig. 78. *Postural deformity after right thoracoplasty.*

2 Resistance with proprioceptive neuromuscular facilitation techniques can be used to improve arm movements.
3 Retraction of the scapulae.
4 Additional neck movements are included, side-flexion towards the operation side only, forward flexion and rotation.

The exercises are gradually progressed with the patient performing them sitting upright, then standing. Trunk forward flexion and side-flexion may be started after about 5 days.

Breathing exercises may be discontinued after 1 week if there are no pulmonary complications, but postural exercises are progressed and continued until the patient is discharged from hospital. A good posture can often be maintained when standing still, but many patients need to give attention to their posture when walking. When discharged from hospital, the patient is advised to continue his exercises and posture correction for 3 months after the date of his operation. If practical, the patient should attend occasionally for assessment and correction of posture.

Surgery for diaphragmatic hernia, achalasia of the cardia (Heller's operation), oesophagectomy, ruptured oesophagus

The same principles of physiotherapy before and after surgery apply to these conditions, but where there is any possibility of reflux, the patient is not treated in the head down position. Humidification may assist clearance of bronchial secretions if the patient is dehydrated.

A lateral thoracotomy through the 6th or 7th intercostal space is used and these lower incisions are usually more painful than the higher ones. Adequate pain control is essential and emphasis must be given to unilateral lower thoracic expansion exercises. Following surgery for diaphragmatic hernia, coughing should not be forced during the first few days.

Patients undergoing surgery of the oesophagus may have a left thoraco-abdominal incision. Effective pain control must be obtained and clearance of bronchial secretions is easier when the surgeon avoids the use of a nasogastric tube. The patient is nursed with the head elevated to at least 30° to prevent regurgitation of the gastric juices.

Correction of pectus excavatum and pectus carinatum

Pectus excavatum or funnel chest and pectus carinatum or pigeon chest are deformities of bone and cartilage of the thorax. With pectus excavatum there is marked depression of the sternum, the xiphoid region moving inwards on inspiration. Pectus carinatum is a deformity where the sternum projects forwards.

The genesis of the deformity is most commonly said to be uncoordinated growth of the ribs owing to a failure of the centres of ossification. If the lower ribs grow more rapidly than the upper ribs, length is provided by displacement of the sternum. This is usually backwards owing to the pull of the diaphragm, pectus excavatum, but may be forwards, pectus carinatum (Ravitch 1983).

Many people with a mild degree of the deformity are symptom free, but it may be corrected surgically if it is causing cardio-respiratory or cosmetic problems. Surgical correction consists of subperichondrial excision of the prominent costal cartilages, detachment of the xiphoid and its re-attachment at a higher level on the sternum. Various surgical techniques are used to hold the sternum forward after excision of the deformed cartilage and rib. A submammary or midsternal incision is used.

Pre-operatively bilateral lower thoracic expansion exercises are practised. Unilateral expansion exercises may produce an uneven pull on the surgical correction. Post-operatively, after recovering from anaesthesia, the patient is usually nursed as upright as possible, well supported by pillows. Some surgeons prefer the patient to lie flat for 24 hours. Breathing exercises should be practised immediately post-operatively. Arm and shoulder girdle exercises, trunk movements, posture correction and ambulation are started as soon as permission is given by the surgeon.

Thymectomy

Thymectomy is performed for the removal of thymoma often associated with myasthenia gravis. The incision is usually a high median sternotomy.

The basic principles of pre- and post-operative physiotherapy apply, but patients with myasthenia gravis become easily fatigued and the physiotherapist should take care not to tire them. If possible, treatment should be given soon after the administration of neostigmine (or another of the anticholinesterase group of drugs).

Some myasthenic patients require ventilation post-operatively and often suffer from excess secretions which occur as a side-effect of neostigmine. Prolonged treatment cannot be tolerated and occasionally it may be necessary to cease treatment before the chest has been completely cleared in order to prevent fatigue (p. 109).

CARDIAC SURGERY IN ADULTS

Most open heart operations are performed through a median sternotomy. These include coronary artery vein grafts, valve replacements, valve annuloplasty, open mitral or pulmonary valvotomy, closure of atrial or ventricular septal defect, total correction of Fallot's tetralogy, excision of ventricular or aortic aneurysm, removal of cardiac myxoma. Pulmonary embolectomy is included since cardiopulmonary bypass is also necessary for this operation.

Sometimes a submammary incision is used for cosmetic reasons for open heart surgery in young female patients.

For closed heart operations a lateral thoracotomy is used. These include ligation of patent ductus arteriosus and excision of coarctation of the aorta.

A median sternotomy, or possibly bilateral anterior thoracotomy, is used for pericardiectomy.

The physiotherapist should know which incision the surgeon will use for each patient in order that emphasis can be given to exercises that will be most important during the post-operative period. Following anaesthesia and surgery there is a fall in functional residual capacity (FRC) and breathing exercises are important.

With cardiac patients treatment must be adapted to the individual's condition. A strict routine must not be followed and the patient must not be exhausted. Pre-operative training is as important as for patients undergoing pulmonary surgery and should be started as early as possible.

Aims of physiotherapy following cardiac surgery

1 To preserve adequate ventilation.
2 To assist removal of excess secretions to minimize the occurrence of atelectasis.
3 To assist the circulation in the legs and to help prevent post-operative venous thrombosis.
4 To maintain mobility of the shoulders, shoulder girdle and spine.
5 To prevent postural deformity.
6 To restore exercise tolerance.

PRE-OPERATIVE TRAINING

1 Explanation to the patient

Explanation by the physiotherapist, in order to gain the patient's confidence and cooperation, is similar to that described for pulmonary surgery (p. 81).

The importance of maintaining adequate ventilation of the lungs by breathing exercises and the clearance of excess secretions from the airways must be explained. Reassurance should be given that breathing exercises, huffing, coughing and coughing and moving around in bed will do no harm to the stitches, drainage tubes or operation site.

A member of the medical staff should tell the patient about the operation including the position of drainage tubes, intravenous drip, nasogastric tube, urinary catheter, electrocardiograph leads, the possibility of an endotracheal tube and the use of a ventilator for a few hours postoperatively. The patient should be warned that if he wakes up with an endotracheal tube in place speaking will be temporarily impossible, but the staff will understand his requirements.

2 Removal of secretions

The majority of patients about to undergo cardiac surgery do not have excess bronchial secretions. Some patients with severe mitral valve disease or longstanding pulmonary hypertension may develop associated chronic obstructive lung disease and assistance with removal of secretions is required. In the early stage of cardiac disease the patient may have a persistent dry cough or expectorate frothy white sputum. This is not a physiotherapy problem.

If a patient has a cold or other respiratory tract infection, surgery should be postponed until the chest is clear.

If a chronic bronchitic is to have cardiac surgery he will need assistance to clear excess secretions from his airways. A modified form of postural drainage (p. 29) should be used. Care should be taken not to cause undue fatigue or dyspnoea.

The head-down postural drainage position should not be used for cardiac patients before or after surgery unless specifically requested by the surgeon.

This position causes an increase in venous return to the heart and an increase in atrial pressures.

3 Breathing control

Breathing control allows the patient to return to the normal pattern of breathing between the more active breathing exercises and following huffing and coughing. It may assist the loosening of secretions in the lower zones of the lungs. The patient is encouraged to relax the upper chest and shoulder girdle and to breathe gently with the lower chest.

4 Breathing exercises

For patients having a median sternotomy, expansion of the lower thorax will be inhibited after surgery and unilateral lower thoracic expansion of both sides of the chest should be practised in the half-lying position. Expansion for the side of the incision must be emphasized when a lateral thoracotomy is to be used.

Holding full inspiration for 3 seconds helps to increase aeration of the alveoli (Ward et al. 1966). This should be repeated four times before returning to breathing control. Longer periods of thoracic expansion exercises may lead to hyper ventilation, but the cycle can be repeated several times.

Pre-operatively the patient should be encouraged to practise these exercises. He should understand that for the first 2 or 3 days after the operation he should practise breathing exercises for at least a few minutes every hour that he is awake in addition to the visits by the physiotherapist.

5 The forced expiration technique and coughing

Effective huffing and coughing are taught as for pulmonary surgery (p. 82). The physiotherapist should show the patient how she will support the chest over the incision and how he can support it himself. For a median sternotomy the patient can hold his hands directly over the front of the sternum (fig. 79) or fold his arms across the chest giving lateral support as well as pressure from the forearms anteriorly. Alternatively he can hold a pillow against the anterior part of his chest. For a lateral incision the arm of the unaffected side is placed across the front of the chest, the hand giving pressure just below the incision, the other elbow giving pressure inwards to the chest wall (fig. 72).

6 Foot and leg exercises

All patients are taught simple foot and ankle exercises and knee flexion and extension in order to assist the circulation and help prevent post-operative venous thrombosis. The importance of practising

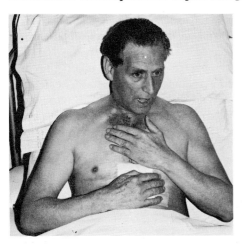

Fig. 79. *Median sternotomy supported by patient.*

these movements several times during every waking hour after surgery should be stressed.

7 Posture, shoulder girdle and arm movements

The habitual posture of the patient is noted pre-operatively and his range of arm movements. Those patients having a median sternotomy are unlikely to have difficulty with shoulder movements after surgery, but the shoulder girdle may become stiff and many patients tend to adopt a slightly kyphotic posture. Shoulder shrugging and 'shrug-circling' are useful exercises and can be practised briefly pre-operatively.

Patients having a lateral thoracotomy need arm and shoulder girdle exercises and postural correction similar to those undergoing pulmonary surgery (p. 83).

8 Pre-operative observations

During pre-operative instruction the physiotherapist should note the patient's normal chest movement, his exercise tolerance, and his habitual sleeping position. Reassurance may be necessary if the patient is required to lie flat during the post-operative period.

POST-OPERATIVE TREATMENT

Before treatment the physiotherapist must read the operation notes and the report of the patient's post-operative progress. Several observations must be made:
1 Respiration: is the patient being artificially ventilated? If not, what is the respiratory rate?

2 Level of consciousness: is the patient alert and fully responsive? Has he moved all his limbs to command since the operation?

3 Colour: is the patient cyanosed?

4 Blood pressure: has it been stable since the operation?

5 Pulse and temperature.

6 ECG: has the cardiac rhythm been stable, or have there been arrhythmias?

7 Pacemaker: is the heart being artificially paced?

8 Intra-aortic balloon pump: is this being used to assist the cardiac output?

9 Drugs: are drugs required to maintain a reasonable blood pressure? What time was the last dose of analgesic given?

10 Drains: where were the drainage tubes inserted at operation? Was the pleural cavity on either side of the chest opened?

11 Drainage: has there been excessive bleeding from any drain site?

12 Blood gas results: is the arterial oxygen tension unduly low or the carbon dioxide level unduly high?

13 Chest radiograph.

14 Auscultation: are the breath sounds satisfactory? Are there any areas of bronchial breathing? It is important to listen to the chest before and after treatment.

15 Sputum: what colour sputum and what quantity has (a) been sucked from the endotracheal tube if ventilated, or (b) been expectorated by the patient?

16 Urine output: has the patient been passing urine since the operation?

Observations of this nature should be made by the physiotherapist before every treatment and any change in the general condition should be considered.

DAY OF OPERATION

If the patient is not on a ventilator, breathing exercises and breathing control can be started on the day of the operation (provided the cardiovascular system is stable) as soon as he is conscious enough to cooperate. After breathing exercises attempts at huffing and coughing should be made.

FIRST AND SECOND DAYS AFTER OPERATION

Physiotherapy will probably be necessary three or four times during the day. The length of treatment should be modified according to the patient's condition and should not cause undue fatigue.

1 Ventilator treatment

Many patients undergoing open heart surgery receive intermittent positive pressure ventilation via an endotracheal tube for a few hours or during the first post-operative night. Endotracheal suction is carried out regularly by the nursing staff and most patients do not require physiotherapy until after the endotracheal tube has been removed by the anaesthetist.

If the patient needs to remain on a mechanical ventilator during the first post-operative day it is likely that his cardiovascular state is unstable. Effective endotracheal suction is probably adequate to maintain reasonably clear airways until his general condition will tolerate more active physiotherapy.

Manual hyperinflation and chest vibrations are contra-indicated if the cardiac output is poor, but if excess secretions are present that cannot be cleared by suction alone, the physiotherapist may give gentle vibrations in time with the expiratory phase of the ventilator.

A few patients require mechanical ventilation for a longer period and the physiotherapy techniques used to clear bronchial secretions will depend on the cardiovascular state of the patient. Manual hyperinflation can cause a drop in cardiac output, fall in blood pressure and sometimes a drop in Pao_2 (Gormezano & Branthwaite 1972a). It is the treatment of choice if there is no contra-indication (p. 112) in the presence of well-defined areas of localized atelectasis and where excess secretions cannot be cleared by chest vibrations with the ventilator (p. 113).

2 Breathing control and breathing exercises

If the patient is not being artificially ventilated, breathing control and breathing exercises should be carried out. Those who have been ventilated should also start breathing exercises once the endotracheal tube has been removed. The patient should be sitting up in bed with the whole back supported by pillows, so that lower chest movements are not inhibited.

Techniques should include:
(a) Breathing control.
(b) Unilateral lower thoracic expansion for both sides of the chest with a 3-second hold at full inspiration.

If there is a median sternotomy, expansion of both sides of the chest (unilaterally) must be encouraged. If a pleural drain is *in situ*, pain may limit movement and emphasis should be given to expand that side of the chest. With a lateral thoracotomy, emphasis is given to expansion of the incision side.

If pain is severely limiting the respiratory excursion, the physiotherapist should treat the patient after an analgesic has been administered.

The patient should be reminded to practise breathing exercises at least every hour that he is awake.

3 The forced expiration technique and coughing

Effective huffing and coughing, as taught pre-operatively, must be encouraged with the chest firmly supported. The patient often finds it easier to huff and cough when sitting forward in bed away from the pillows. Care must be taken to avoid displacing any drips or wires attached to the patient.

In the absence of heart failure or co-existent lung disease, there are likely to be fewer secretions in the airways than after lung surgery.

If the breath sounds are satisfactory and the chest radiograph does not show atelectasis, the patient will be treated in the sitting position. If there is atelectasis or there are secretions in the lungs that the patient is unable to clear, he should be positioned on his side as flat as he can tolerate. Breathing exercises should be carried out, followed by huffing and coughing. If assistance with clearance of secretions is necessary in patients in acute pulmonary oedema or with cardiac arrhythmias they should not lie flat, but may tolerate a high side-lying position.

The foot of the bed should not be raised for postural drainage of a cardiac patient unless it is specifically ordered by the surgeon (p. 100).

Physiotherapy with periodic continuous positive airway pressure (PCPAP) or intermittent positive pressure breathing (IPPB) can help to re-expand atelectatic areas and loosen secretions (p. 129 &

p. 120). This is often effective in the sitting position, but may be used in side-lying if necessary.

4 Foot and leg exercises

The exercises taught pre-operatively should be practised and the patient should be reminded to do these movements 5–10 times every hour that he is awake.

If an intra-aortic balloon pump is in use, bilateral foot exercises and hip and knee flexion on the unaffected side are given. Hip and knee flexion on the side of the intra-aortic balloon pump may not be given until it has been removed.

5 Shoulder movements

With a lateral thoracotomy it is important to start arm movements on the first post-operative day. With a median sternotomy these need not be started until the second day.

6 Moving in bed

Initially the patient should be lifted by two assistants into a comfortable, well-supported position in bed. Pressure on both arms should be avoided during the first 3 post-operative days. A patient who is not overweight uses the technique of shifting his pelvis backwards one side at a time.

THIRD DAY ONWARDS

Treatment following cardiac surgery must be adapted to the individual patient's condition. The patient will start to sit out of bed from 24 hours after surgery according to his progress and the surgeon's instructions. Walking around the ward may be started as soon as the second or third post-operative day.

The number of times a day that physiotherapy is required depends on the patient's condition and it can probably be reduced to one or two treatments per day by the fourth or fifth day.

Treatment should include:
1 Breathing control and breathing exercises (as above). The patient can be positioned in side-lying if expansion is limited or breath sounds reduced. Bilateral lower thoracic expansion can be included.
2 Huffing and coughing, if secretions are present in the lungs.
3 Foot and leg exercises are given while the patient is confined to bed. These can be discontinued when he is fully mobile.
4 Arm and shoulder girdle exercises.
5 Postural correction and gentle trunk exercises if necessary.
6 Walking up stairs can usually be started about 5–6 days from the time of operation; progress may be slower with patients who have had valve replacements. This will depend on the instructions of the individual surgeon. After cardiac surgery most patients find climbing stairs much less exhausting than pre-operatively, but on occasions it is helpful to teach breathing control with walking on the stairs.

Treatment must be modified if any complications occur.

BEFORE DISCHARGE

Thoracic expansion, shoulder mobility and posture should have returned to normal. The patient should be increasing his exercise tolerance.

The patient should continue breathing exercises for about 2 weeks following the operation, although he will probably be discharged after 10 days.

If he still has excess bronchial secretions when discharged from hospital the patient is advised to continue his physiotherapy at home until his chest is clear.

He is encouraged to take daily exercise, walking about 200 metres on the level at the time of discharge and gradually increasing this distance. By 3 weeks postoperatively he may be achieving a walk of at least 1 km and 4 km daily at 6 weeks.

Rotational movements and heavy lifting must be avoided for 6 weeks as it takes this period for the sternum to heal. The patient should not drive a car for 6–8 weeks and competitive sports should not be played for 3 months although swimming and golf are allowed after 8 weeks.

Some patients benefit from attending a cardiac rehabilitation class to increase their confidence and exercise tolerance. It is usual to start these classes 6–8 weeks after cardiac surgery.

COMPLICATIONS OF CARDIAC SURGERY

Following cardiac surgery, the patient will be continuously assessed by the medical staff, complications will be detected and appropriate treatment prescribed. Such complications include cardiac failure, tamponade (compression of the heart by fluid or clot in the pericardium), haemorrhage, arrhythmias, and fluid and electrolyte imbalance. Other complications that particularly influence the treatment given by the physiotherapist are as follows:

1 Pulmonary oedema

Pulmonary oedema should be suspected if there is a drop in urine output, a raised central venous pressure and an increase in pulmonary secretions. Copious frothy sputum may be an early indication of pulmonary oedema. This may be white at first, becoming pink if the condition is allowed to progress.

If a patient develops acute pulmonary oedema and is being artificially ventilated, physiotherapy should be temporarily discontinued until the condition has been treated. If the patient is breathing independently, he may require assistance to expectorate the excess secretions, but medical treatment (diuretics, etc.) will be required to relieve the condition.

2 Use of the intra-aortic balloon pump

The intra-aortic balloon pump can provide mechanical circulatory assistance when there is poor left ventricular function, or myocardial infarction resulting from low cardiac output or when the patient is in cardiogenic shock. The effect of the intra-aortic balloon pump is to increase systemic arterial pressure and to increase blood flow through the coronary arteries improving myocardial oxygenation (Cleeton 1978).

It may be used pre-operatively and post-operatively where myocardial function is poor. The balloon is inserted via the femoral artery into the descending aorta and is connected to an external balloon and pump. The patient is nursed with the head elevated no more than 30° to avoid occlusion of the catheter in the femoral artery. Hip and knee movements must not be encouraged for the affected leg. When the patient is turned on his side, care must be taken that the hip is flexed no more than 30°. Apart from restriction in positioning for treatment, chest physiotherapy is given according to assessment of the patient. The physiotherapist must be careful to avoid placing her hands over or near the electrocardiograph (ECG) electrodes because the ECG is the trigger to which the balloon pump responds. Any disturbance, for example vibratory shaking of the chest, may interfere with the synchronization of the pump.

3 Pleural effusion

Expansion exercises must be practised in order to prevent restriction of chest movement due to thickening of the pleura. Aspiration may be needed for large effusions.

4 Breakdown of the sternal sutures

If the sternal suture line is breaking down due to infection, the patient's temperature may be raised, there may be oozing from the wound and possibly a noticeable 'click' when the patient coughs or breathes deeply. Firm support must be given to the chest during huffing and coughing, both by the staff and also by the patient when he is coughing independently. Extra support may be given using a towel or wide strap. Care must be taken to prevent straining the suture line when the patient turns over in bed.

5 Neurological damage

Occasionally during cardiac surgery the brain may be damaged by embolism or anoxia. The physiotherapist must treat any form of paralysis that occurs and rehabilitate the patient as soon as possible. The patient's cardiac state may limit the form of rehabilitation.

6 Renal failure

Another rare complication of cardiac surgery is renal failure. Occasionally peritoneal dialysis will have to be instituted. Breathing exercises are particularly important to maintain function of the lung bases. Physiotherapy should be carried out during the period when the peritoneum is almost empty, in order to allow maximal basal expansion. Movement of the diaphragm will be limited when the abdomen is filled with fluid and the patient will find it uncomfortable if physiotherapy is given at this time. This also applies to physiotherapy if the dialysed patient is being artificially ventilated.

PROBLEMS WITH INDIVIDUAL CARDIAC OPERATIONS

Resection of coarctation of the aorta

During the first 10 days after resection of coarctation of the aorta there are likely to be episodes of hypertension. The reason for this phenomenon is unknown, but if it occurs it could put a strain on the aortic suture line. The physiotherapist should be aware of the possibility and modify the treatment to avoid increasing the hypertension. It may be contra-indicated to lie the patient flat, even if bronchial secretions are present.

Pulmonary embolectomy

Pulmonary embolectomy may be performed for massive pulmonary embolism. Post-operative physiotherapy should be similar to that for open heart surgery, but pulmonary dysfunction is especially common owing to the presence of small infarcts. The patient is likely to be cyanosed and will expectorate dark brown, blood stained sputum.

Manual hyperinflation with chest vibration may be indicated while the patient is artificially ventilated.

Pericardiectomy

Following this operation patients may be troubled with excessive amounts of frothy sputum and need encouragement with coughing.

Insertion of pacemaker

Pacemakers are inserted for the treatment of heart block and are usually inserted under local anaesthesia using angiography. If a general anaesthetic is used the patient should be assessed and treated by the physiotherapist if necessary.

TRANSPLANTATION

Heart transplantation

Patients receiving a heart transplant require pre- and post-operative physiotherapy similar to treatment for open heart surgery. Many of these patients will have been ill for a long period and will have been leading a restricted life. They require emphasis on improving exercise tolerance and muscle power and need to gain confidence to return to a more normal independent life.

The patient is usually extubated after a few hours of intermittent positive pressure ventilation and starts breathing exercises and leg exercises in bed an hour after extubation. On the second post-operative day, if his general condition permits, the patient does a few simple leg exercises in standing (each movement three times only at first), knee-bends in a small range from standing, heel raising and standing from sitting. While sitting out of bed the patient starts using exercise pedals for 1 minute (with no added resistance) twice a day. This is progressed by 1 to 2 minutes a day until the fifth day when a programme on an exercise bicycle can be started.

The overall aim is to increase endurance and strength. A programme gradually progressing with time and the resistance for each individual is worked out.

As soon as all intravenous infusions have been discontinued the patient starts walking increasing distances outside his room and by the seventh or eighth post-operative day stair-climbing may be started and a full flight of stairs will probably be achieved before the patient is discharged on the tenth post-operative day. Some patients will have been severely ill pre-operatively and will progress more slowly.

An exercise record card is used in hospital and should be continued at home. The patient is instructed in a gradual progression of exercise, but warned that if he becomes unusually fatigued it is a sign that he is doing too much exercise and should adapt his regimen accordingly. Approximately 6 weeks after surgery the patient may join a rehabilitation class to continue his progressive exercise programme.

It is important that the relatives are aware of the amount of exercise the patient can achieve before he leaves hospital. The relatives need to gain confidence so that they can encourage exercise and independence rather than over-protect the patient.

Immunosuppressant drugs are then

required for the rest of the patient's life and he is warned that his defence mechanisms against infection are lowered. He is advised to avoid contact with people with obvious infections. For the first 24–48 hours post-operatively the patient may be reverse-barrier nursed or if he is intubated for a longer period, barrier nursing may continue until he is extubated.

The physiotherapist must be aware that some of the immunosuppressant drugs may cause a fall in arterial blood pressure. Electrocardiograph, echocardiograph and cardiac biopsy are carried out regularly and if there are any signs of rejection of the transplant, the exercise programme must be stopped until the episode is over.

Heart–lung transplantation

Heart–lung transplantation is carried out for selected patients with end-stage pulmonary or cardiopulmonary disease. The operation was at first limited to those patients with severe irreversible pulmonary vascular disease, but with the improvement of long-term survival the indications for this operation have been extended to include several pulmonary and cardiac disorders (Hakim & Wallwork 1985).

The patients who have a heart–lung transplant have usually been ill for a prolonged period pre-operatively and their post-operative progress is likely to be slower than for the patients undergoing a heart transplant operation.

The principles of treatment are similar, but the heart–lung patients have bilateral pleural drains and emphasis must be given to clearing and maintaining clear lungs. Below the tracheal anastamosis there is denervation and the sensation normally felt with the presence of excess bronchial secretions is lacking.

Lower lateral thoracic expansion exercises are encouraged in side-lying and postural drainage for the lateral segments of the lower lobes is started after 3 or 4 post-operative days and continued twice daily until the patient is discharged. He is advised to continue postural drainage once daily at home as a prophylactic treatment. The patient should be encouraged to listen to the sound of his huff to low lung volume. Detection of secretions by the sound may be helpful in the absence of normal sensation and may make prophylactic postural drainage unnecessary. Progression of leg exercises, bicycling, walking and going up stairs is similar to the programme for patients following a heart transplant.

8 Physiotherapy for patients receiving mechanical ventilation

INTERMITTENT POSITIVE PRESSURE VENTILATION (IPPV)

There are many reasons for patients requiring intermittent positive pressure ventilation (IPPV), but common factors need to be considered before the physiotherapist carries out treatment. The medical records, equipment for ventilation, clinical recordings, observation and examination of the patient provide important information.

1 *The medical records* must be studied for recent investigations and diagnosis, in addition to relevant past medical history.

2 The most recent *chest radiograph* is compared to previous radiographs.

3 Has the patient an *endotracheal or tracheal* tube? Is it a cuffed tube?

4 *Type of ventilation.* Is the patient fully ventilated with IPPV? Is positive end expiratory pressure (PEEP) in use? If the patient is not fully ventilated is he on synchronized intermittent mandatory ventilation (SIMV) or continuous positive airway pressure (CPAP)? Has the mode of ventilation been altered within the last 2 hours? It may be necessary to allow the patient to stabilize before physiotherapy.

5 *The ventilator recordings* are noted: respiratory rate, minute ventilation, airway pressure, PEEP setting if in use, inspired oxygen concentration.

6 *Type of humidification*: Is a vapour condenser humidifier in the circuit or a hot water or nebulizer system?

7 *The arterial blood gas results* are compared with previous results.

8 Is the patient's *blood pressure* adequate and stable?

9 What is the patient's *temperature* and *heart rate*?

10 Is the *urine output* satisfactory?

11 Is the *cardiac rhythm* stable?

12 What *drugs* is the patient receiving? Are cardiovascular support drugs required? Has the patient been sedated or been given analgesics?

13 What is the *level of consciousness* of the patient? If the patient is unconscious, is this due to the underlying condition or is it drug induced?

14 The *colour* of the patient is observed: cyanosis may be an indicator of hypoxaemia, a yellow colour may indicate renal and/or hepatic failure.

15 Is the patient showing signs of peripheral vasoconstriction—is his skin *cold and clammy*? This may be a sign of poor cardiac output.

16 Is the *chest expanding* equally on both sides?

17 Are the *breath sounds* equal on both sides of the chest? Are there bronchial breath sounds or added sounds? Observation of chest movement and auscultation occasionally reveals that the endotracheal tube has slipped beyond the carina and into the right main bronchus.

18 What colour and quantity of *secretions*

have been suctioned from the endotracheal tube?

19 Has the patient any *chest drains in situ?*

The physiotherapist should not only be concerned with the patient's chest condition, but must consider and treat the general condition of the patient as well as remembering the possible feelings and fears that he may have in his unnatural surroundings.

A survey of patients' memories of their experiences in intensive care units (Asbury 1985) revealed that more attention should be given to some aspects of care. Many patients lost perception of time, some ventilated patients were worried at their inability to speak and others would have preferred more information about their treatment. The physiotherapist can help patients by giving frequent explanations of their treatment procedures, reassurance and explanation of the reasons for the inability to speak when a cuffed endotracheal tube is in place and a constant reminder of time (Innocenti

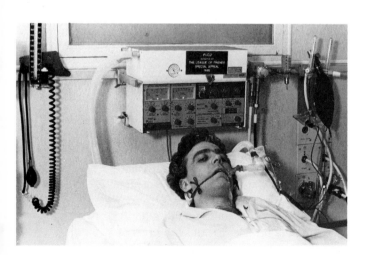

Fig. 80. *Mechanical ventilation via an endotracheal tube.*

1986). These explanations should be given even if the physiotherapist thinks that the patient may not be able to hear or comprehend.

When a patient is being mechanically ventilated via an endotracheal tube (fig. 80) or tracheostomy there are several factors, apart from the underlying disease, that predispose to excess bronchial secretions and chest infection. These include:

1 The inability to cough effectively.

2 The absence of the normal deep sigh mechanism.

3 The presence of a tube which irritates the mucus membrane.

4 The tendency for drying and crusting of secretions and infection, due to bypass of the upper respiratory tract.

By regular turning of the patient if this is not contra-indicated, adequate humidification and tracheal suction and care in maintaining sterile precautions, problems of excess secretions can be kept to a minimum. However, assistance with removal of secretions is often required and the most effective method is known as *manual hyperinflation with chest vibration.* It is often termed 'bag squeezing', but this name does not infer the all important type of inflation that is given (Clement & Hübsch 1968).

Manual hyperinflation with chest vibration

The patient is positioned on his side if possible and the endotracheal tube or tracheostomy tube, is disconnected from the ventilator and connected to a manual inflation bag. The position chosen for treatment will depend on the results of auscultation and the chest radiograph. One person, often an anaesthetist, squeezes the bag inflating the chest with a slow deep inspiration which promotes aeration of the alveoli. After holding the full inspiration momentarily the bag is released quickly, to allow a high expiratory flow rate. The physiotherapist has her hands on the side of the lower rib cage and starts to compress the chest just at the end of the inspiratory period, fractionally before the bag is released. This accurate synchronization between the two operators is essential to produce the best effect. The chest compression, reinforcing the high expiratory flow rate from the bag, assists movement of the secretions in the periphery of the lung towards the main airways (fig. 81).

Approximately six deep breaths with chest vibrations are given and this is followed by suction. Suction should also precede hyperinflation if there are audible secretions in the large airways. If the patient is conscious and able to cooperate, he is encouraged to attempt to cough actively when the suction catheter has been inserted and at the same time the physiotherapist vibrates the chest to assist removal of secretions (fig. 82).

The whole procedure is probably repeated two or three times with the physiotherapist vibrating over the basal area. When that area is clear, the middle and upper areas of the chest are treated if secretions are present.

The number of times per day that treatment is performed depends both on the condition of the patient's chest and on his general condition. It may be necessary to carry it out every 2 hours or even hourly, or it may only be required once or twice a day. Where possible, treatment should be timed to coincide with the nurses turning regimen to avoid unnecessary discomfort to the patient.

Some form of sedation and/or analgesia

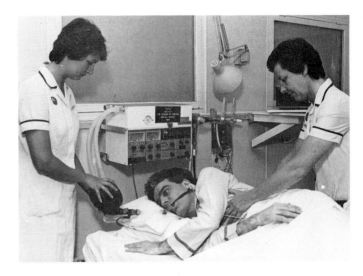

Fig. 81. *Manual hyperinflation with chest vibrations.*

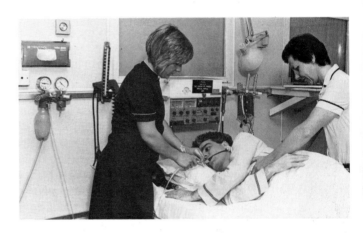

Fig. 82. *Endotracheal suction with chest vibrations.*

is often necessary before treatment or treatment may be timed to coincide with sedation already prescribed. The analgesic effect produced by a mixture of 50% nitrous oxide and 50% oxygen (Entonox, p. 140) may occasionally be helpful. Manual hyperinflation with Entonox may be desirable during the phase of weaning from the ventilator when the sedative effects of other drugs may be undesirable.

Manual hyperinflation for the patient who is alert and taking some breaths spontaneously should be carefully synchronized with the patient's breathing.

If the secretions are thick, it is often helpful to insert 2 or 3 ml of normal saline (0.9%) into the trachea before hyperinflating the chest. The saline will go into the most dependent bronchi, and should therefore be inserted before positioning the patient to drain the affected area.

Suction of the intubated patient must be carried out with a sterile technique using gloves. A suitable sized catheter is inserted into the endotracheal or tracheostomy tube to reach just beyond the end of the tube. Theoretically the diameter of the catheter should not be more than half the diameter of the tube through which it is passing. A Y-connection should be used between the catheter and suction apparatus and suction should not be applied until the catheter is fully inserted. The catheter is withdrawn using a rotating action between the finger and thumb so that all available secretions are aspirated. The duration of suction should not exceed 15 seconds. The same catheter should not be used again.

If difficulty is experienced in passing the catheter down an endotracheal tube, it may be helpful to extend the patient's neck or turn his head to one side. The flexed position of the neck may cause slight kinking of the tube. It may also help to instil more saline immediately prior to suction.

Where even minimal trauma would be dangerous because of a stitch line in the trachea or at the carina, it may be necessary to use cushion-tip catheters which are specially designed to prevent mucosal damage.

A specimen of bronchial secretions is often required for laboratory investigations. A 'trap specimen' is collected by means of a special specimen container with a catheter attached, connected to the suction apparatus.

If the patient has a vapour condenser humidifier in the ventilator circuit it must be changed every 24 hours, or immediately if it becomes soiled with bronchial secretions.

Equipment for inflation

An anaesthetic rebreathing bag is usually used for manual hyperinflation. Alternatively the self re-inflating Ambu bag may be used. It is important that the system provides a good elastic recoil when the bag is released. A 2-litre bag is normally used for adults.

Most commonly a mixture of air with a controlled quantity of added oxygen is used for hyperinflation. Provided that there is an adequate gas flow of 10–15 litres/minute, it should not be necessary to use a Waters CO_2 absorbing canister in the circuit as this can be cumbersome and heavy. Occasionally Entonox is used as the hyperinflation gas.

Contra-indications to manual hyperinflation

Hyperinflation with chest vibrations can in some cases produce a fall in cardiac output and a lowering of the arterial oxygen tension (Gormezano & Branthwaite 1972a). It should only be undertaken when there is some valid indication and with the agreement of the medical staff.

The following conditions contra-indicate hyperinflation:

1 Unstable cardiovascular condition such

as low cardiac output and some cardiac arrhythmias.

2 Severe hypoxaemia when few bronchial secretions are present, for example adult respiratory distress syndrome (p. 117).

3 Acute pulmonary oedema. Tracheal suction can increase pulmonary oedema, but the proximal secretions can be removed by suction as necessary. Physiotherapy should be postponed until the pulmonary oedema has been controlled by medical treatment.

4 Air leak. If there is a pneumothorax, surgical emphysema or an intercostal tube in place with a severe air leak, hyperinflation is likely to be contra-indicated. It will not be suitable for a patient with a lung condition predisposing to pneumothorax, for example emphysema, cystic fibrosis, irreversible fibrosis following severe 'shock lung syndrome'.

5 Severe bronchospasm. Where bronchospasm is the main problem, hyperinflation is not indicated until this has been relieved, for example acute asthma.

6 Haemoptysis.

Alternative method of chest treatment

If hyperinflation is contra-indicated, but physiotherapy is required to assist removal of secretions, an alternative method may be used. The chest is vibrated in time with the expiratory phase of the ventilator instead of giving any extra inflation. The patient can be positioned, saline instilled and suction and coughing performed in the same way as previously described.

Limb movements

Unconscious or paralysed patients should have passive movements to all their limbs.

Active movements should be encouraged whenever possible.

For patients with neurological conditions, the basic principles for positioning, nursing and subsequent rehabilitation should be applied.

Weaning from a ventilator

Weaning from the ventilator is started when the patient's condition has improved sufficiently and should be carried out under the supervision of the anaesthetist. The criteria usually required before a patient can be successfully weaned from a ventilator are: a clear chest radiograph, minimal bronchial secretions, normal blood gases on 40% oxygen or less and a functioning gastrointestinal tract.

A patient who is intubated and ventilated for a few hours, for example following cardiac surgery, will probably be extubated after a short period of spontaneous ventilation through the endotracheal tube.

For a patient requiring IPPV for a longer period there are several methods from which the anaesthetist can choose to assist the patient during the weaning phase from the ventilator. The ventilator controls may be altered to allow the patient to breathe with synchronized intermittent mandatory ventilation (SIMV) or continuous positive airway pressure (CPAP), or the patient may be transferred to a pressure-cycled ventilator which he can self-trigger.

Alternatively the patient may start by breathing without the ventilator for short periods, gradually lengthening the time according to the anaesthetist's instructions. With all weaning methods there should be careful monitoring of respiratory and pulse rates and arterial blood gases. The patient is reconnected to the ventilator if there are signs of respiratory distress.

For patients breathing independently through a tracheostomy tube, humidification is essential to prevent bronchial secretions becoming thick and tenacious. An attachment to the tracheostomy tube will provide humidified air with the appropriate amount of additional oxygen.

Breathing exercises should be started during this stage to re-educate active use of the respiratory muscles. The patient should be encouraged to cough voluntarily instead of relying entirely on the stimulation of the suction catheter.

When the patient is breathing independently for several hours in the day, physiotherapy will probably comprise active breathing exercises in the side-lying position with vibrations, huffing and tracheal suction. Manual hyperinflation can be continued if necessary, but this should be stopped as soon as the patient is able to huff and cough effectively so that he can manage without assistance once the tube has been removed.

Patients who are weaned on a pressure-cycled ventilator, for example the Bird Mark 7, may be more comfortable with physiotherapy by self-triggered hyperinflation from the Bird instead of manual hyperinflation from a rebreathing bag. The pressure on the ventilator can be increased to give a hyperinflation, or the nurse can be requested to press the manual trigger, after the patient has triggered the ventilator, to give an inspiratory plateau. With both methods, chest vibrations or shaking are given during expiration.

A patient with a cuffed tracheostomy tube will progress to a speaking tube. This may be an uncuffed, fenestrated, silver tube from which the inner cannula can be removed when the patient is spontaneously breathing. An inner tube with a speaking flap allows air to pass through the vocal cords.

The Shiley, fenestrated, low pressure, cuffed tracheostomy tube combines features for IPPV, or spontaneous ventilation with a cuffed or speaking tube. If the inner cannula is removed and the decannulation cannula is occluding the lumen of the outer cannula, it is essential that the cuff is fully deflated to allow the patient to self-ventilate adequately. With fenestrated tubes the inner cannula should be re-inserted for suction to avoid the catheter passing through the fenestration and causing mucosal trauma.

After removal of the tube, the dressing covering the tracheostomy should be as airtight as possible, but it is still necessary to teach the patient to hold the site of the tracheostomy firmly while coughing (fig. 83). If there is an air leak, some of the secretions and air are blown out through

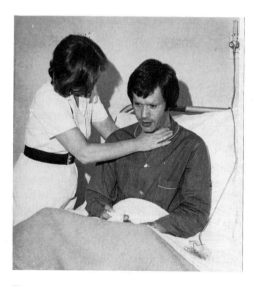

Fig. 83. *Coughing after removal of tracheostomy tube.*

the incision instead of being expectorated from the mouth and the full force of the cough is wasted.

For the first 48 hours after removal of a tracheostomy tube, it is often necessary to increase the frequency of treatments to assist clearance of secretions. At this stage, the assistance of IPPB with physiotherapy may help the patient to overcome a critical period (p. 120).

VARIATIONS OF TREATMENT WITH SPECIFIC CONDITIONS

1 Post-cardiac surgery

The indication for treatment by manual hyperinflation with chest vibration depends on the volume of bronchial secretions present and on the cardio-vascular state of the patient (p. 102).

If treatment is indicated the patient may need to remain supine. With one hand supporting the incision, gentle vibrations are given to the side of the chest using the other hand. If the patient is treated in side-lying and has had a median sternotomy, care must be taken to avoid giving too much pressure to the lateral chest wall. The hands are placed more posteriorly than laterally and during suction the incision should be supported by one hand and forearm, while vibrating the posterior aspect of the chest wall with the other hand.

The physiotherapist must be aware of any change in the ECG pattern or colour of the patient. Development of cool, clammy skin may indicate peripheral vasoconstriction and a fall in cardiac output. The blood pressure should be taken during treatment if it has been unstable. Treatment periods should be brief as there is the danger of causing a fall in Pao_2.

2 Post-pulmonary surgery

If a patient requires IPPV following pulmonary surgery, physiotherapy with manual hyperinflation may be helpful. It can, if necessary, be combined with postural drainage for the appropriate area. It may be contra-indicated if there is a large air leak or any sign of surgical emphysema.

3 Acute exacerbation of chronic bronchitis

It is rare that a patient with an acute exacerbation of chronic bronchitis requires intubation and ventilation, but should this occur there may be copious thick secretions at the lung bases. Initially, vigorous physiotherapy will be needed at least every 2 hours. The patient can be positioned for drainage of the affected lobes before and during treatment. The chest shaking can be more energetic than with surgical patients, as there is no painful incision.

4 Asthma

Occasionally a patient suffering from asthma may be intubated and ventilated. The small airways may be plugged with bronchial casts, but manual hyperinflation and chest vibrations tend to aggravate bronchospasm and should not be started until the secretions begin to liquefy and bronchodilatation starts to occur. Some physicians prescribe 2 ml of normal saline (0·9%) to be instilled into the endotracheal tube every 15 minutes by the nursing staff to assist in loosening the bronchial casts.

Physiotherapy is probably not indicated until the patient has been extubated, but if manual hyperinflation is used, 2–3 ml of normal saline is instilled before each group of inflations. If treatment is found to aggravate bronchospasm, it should be discontinued until the patient's condition has improved. It is often helpful to give a bronchodilator before treatment. A ventilator suitable for IPPB, (p. 120) with a bronchodilator in the nebulizer can be connected to the endotracheal tube.

5 Respiratory muscle paralysis

If the respiratory muscles are paralysed, for example by acute polyneuritis or poliomyelitis, IPPV may be necessary. Manual hyperinflation is a suitable method of treatment, but rib springing is often a more effective means of moving the secretions than chest vibrations in the paralysed patient. To perform rib springing the physiotherapist gives pressure throughout expiration and then increases her pressure squeezing the air out of the chest at the end of expiration, before releasing her hands quickly to allow expansion to occur during inspiration.

6 Tetanus

Many patients are heavily sedated with diazepam (Valium) and artificially ventilated. Additional sedation should be given prior to physiotherapy and if there are any signs of muscle spasm, treatment should be temporarily discontinued until further sedation has been administered. Occasionally patients are therapeutically paralysed. Tetanus patients tend to have an unstable autonomic nervous system, fluctuations in blood pressure may occur and treatment may have to be adapted.

Physiotherapy includes appropriate postural drainage with manual hyperinflation and chest compression. There is often hypersecretion of mucus and areas of lobar collapse may occur. Treatments may need to be carried out every 2 hours in the early stages of the disease. Passive movements of the limbs should be given regularly and care should be taken to position them comfortably.

7 Crushed chest

If a patient with a crushed chest requires IPPV, chest shaking to the affected side is usually contra-indicated. Positioning of the patient combined with manual hyperinflation may be used with caution provided that an intercostal drain has been inserted. If there is contusion of the underlying lung there will be thick, blood-stained secretions and extra saline instilled into the endotracheal or tracheostomy tube may be indicated. Support of the affected area of the chest should be given during attempts at huffing and coughing and during suction.

Adequate analgesia before physiotherapy is essential. The patient may have an intercostal nerve block to relieve the pain or Entonox may be indicated for manual hyperinflation.

8 Head injury

Patients with a severe head injury may require IPPV and may benefit from chest physiotherapy, but the neurological state and intracranial pressure (ICP) must be carefully considered.

One method of controlling ICP is by hyperventilation in order to lower the arterial carbon dioxide level ($Pa\text{CO}_2$) which produces vasoconstriction of the cerebral arterioles. A raised $Pa\text{CO}_2$ causes vasodilatation and will cause an increase in ICP. It is important for the physiotherapist to prevent retention of bronchial secretions and atelectasis to avoid an increase in $Pa\text{CO}_2$.

With manual hyperinflation it is likely that the increase in intrathoracic pressure and restriction of venous return will raise the ICP, but the treatment can produce hyperventilation and this will tend to lower the $Pa\text{CO}_2$ and the increase in ICP may not be significant. It is important to note the rate of the ventilator and to squeeze the manual hyperinflation bag at a rate no slower than this. Chest vibrations are given with manual hyperinflation unless the patient has rib fractures.

Analgesics should be given to control pain and sedation given to avoid agitation of the patient as both these factors can increase ICP. Positioning of the patient will be limited by the other injuries sustained. If a flap of bone has been removed, care must be taken to avoid the patient's head resting with pressure on this unprotected area of the brain. The neurosurgeon may permit the head-down postural drainage position despite it causing an increase in ICP. Short treatments of about 5–10 minutes may be undertaken while carefully monitoring the patient.

Normal intracranial pressure is 0–10 mmHg. ICP higher than 25 mmHg will probably contra-indicate physiotherapy, but the benfits of chest treatment have to be balanced against the possibility of increasing ICP. There may be a subdural transducer monitoring ICP, but changes in arterial blood pressure are a useful guide to changes in ICP. If the arterial blood pressure is high, ICP is also high and if chest physiotherapy causes a rise in blood pressure there will also be a rise in ICP.

Endotracheal suction is carried out to remove secretions mobilized by treatment, but suction and coughing both promote a rise in ICP and hyperventilation of the patient with the manual inflation bag following suction will lower the ICP. Suction of the nose and pharynx is necessary if the patient cannot swallow, but if there is a fracture of the base of the skull with a leak of cerebrospinal fluid, nasal suction must be omitted.

To reduce a raised ICP the patient is nursed with his head elevated to 30° and movement of the head away from the neutral position should be avoided. Small changes in the position of the head and neck away from the midline can increase ICP (Shapiro 1975). When the patient is turned on his side, his head should be maintained in alignment throughout the procedure to prevent an increase in ICP (Hough 1986). If the patient remains unconscious, but begins to be weaned from the ventilator, techniques to facilitate respiratory movement patterns are beneficial (Bethune 1975).

Limb movements are carried out passively at first, but progressed according to the individual's condition.

9 Adult respiratory distress syndrome (ARDS)

ARDS is a condition resulting from diverse insults to the lung. It affects the alveoli rather than the airways and usually accompanies or follows a circulatory crisis in patients with previously normal lungs. The diverse conditions which may result in ARDS include trauma with major haemorrhage, blast injury, lung contusion, septicaemia, acute viral pneumonia, fat and amniotic fluid embolism, inhalation of noxious substances, aspiration of gastric contents or near-drowning.

The early pathological changes are interstitial inflammation with haemorrhage and oedema. Increased alveolar-capillary permeability is a feature of ARDS with increased levels of interstitial fluid containing large amounts of protein. Fibrin or hyaline membranes line affected alveoli and eventually a proliferation of fibroblasts leads to interstitial fibrosis.

Clinical features are dyspnoea, tachypnoea, tachycardia and hypoxaemia in spite of high inspired oxygen concentrations. There are scanty physical signs in the chest and at first the chest radiograph is normal. Subsequently it shows extensive 'fluffy' shadows and this may be followed by a complete 'white out' of the lung fields. Pneumothoraces may develop at a later stage when fibrosis occurs.

Most patients require intubation and IPPV and even with the addition of PEEP it is often difficult to maintain adequate arterial oxygen levels.

Physiotherapy with manual hyperinflation is contra-indicated in patients with severe hypoxaemia and few secretions (Branthwaite 1980). If excess bronchial secretions develop physiotherapy may be indicated, but care must be taken to avoid decreasing arterial oxygen levels with treatment, positioning and suction. The risk of pneumothorax developing in the later stages of the condition must be remembered and vibrations with the patient on the ventilator may be indicated in preference to manual hyperinflation.

10 Inhalation burns

Patients with inhalation burns may develop oedema of the upper respiratory tract or stridor and require intubation using a soft nasotracheal tube to maintain an adequate airway. IPPV is necessary if oxygenation is unsatisfactory.

Manual hyperinflation with chest vibrations and postural drainage can be used if excess bronchial secretions or areas of atelectasis are present. Strict aseptic precautions must be used as patients with burns of the respiratory tract are susceptible to infection. Careful suction using catheters causing minimal trauma to the airways should be carried out, to allow tissue healing to proceed.

BRONCHIAL LAVAGE

When there is a tenacious exudate in the periphery of the lungs, either in the terminal bronchioles or alveoli, which is not responsive to the routine methods of removal (for example postural drainage, humidification, IPPB), the procedure known as bronchial lavage is occasionally used. The term bronchial lavage is used for two distinct procedures one involving the instillation of large volumes of solution into the bronchial tree and the other using small volumes of solution.

The procedure involving the larger volumes of fluid is indicated for the treatment of alveolar proteinosis (du Bois *et al.* 1983) and occasionally has been used for intractable attacks of asthma. If the exudate in the periphery of the lungs is allowed to remain, it impairs aeration of the alveoli and inhibits gas transfer.

The aim of bronchial lavage is to flush out as much of the exudate as possible. It is a skilled procedure carried out under general anaesthesia using a double lumen tube. One lung is gradually filled to FRC (functional residual capacity) with warmed buffered electrolyte solution. Further volumes of electrolyte solution are instilled and drained out aiming to keep the volume of the treated lung at FRC or approximately 500 ml above FRC. After up to 20 litres of electrolyte solution have been used, the lung is drained completely using suction and posture. The lung is then reinflated by positive pressure ventilation and a short period of post-treatment ventilatory support is often employed. Bronchopulmonary lavage is more difficult and more dangerous to carry out in the treatment of asthma because the solution drains out of the lungs less easily.

Occasionally following extubation, assisted breathing by use of IPPB and encouragement to cough may be necessary and possibly postural drainage. However, when a few hours of mechanical ventilation are used after the procedure minimal physiotherapy is required because so little fluid remains in the lungs.

The bronchial lavage procedure involving small volumes of solution is carried out using a fibre-optic bronchoscope. This method is sometimes employed in an attempt to remove mucus plugs in bronchopulmonary aspergillosis or asthma. Small quantities (5–10 ml at a time, up to 50–100 ml) of sterile saline are instilled down the centre channel of the bronchoscope. Viscid secretions may be liquefied and removed from the affected bronchial segments.

9 Adjuncts to physiotherapy

INTERMITTENT POSITIVE PRESSURE BREATHING (IPPB)

In the spontaneously breathing patient, intermittent positive pressure breathing (IPPB) is the maintenance of a positive airway pressure throughout inspiration, with airway pressure returning to atmospheric pressure during expiration.

IPPB should not be used 'routinely' but it may be a useful adjunct to treatment when physiotherapy techniques alone cannot produce the desired result.

The effects of IPPB on chronic respiratory patients have been studied, but clinical trials with acute patients are difficult to perform. It is important that the results of studies on chronic patients are not extrapolated to the short-term use of IPPB in acute patients.

Studies of IPPB have shown no long-term benefit in patients with chronic airflow limitation (Intermittent Positive Pressure Breathing Trial Group 1983). Daily periods of IPPB have been shown to improve lung compliance and decrease the work of breathing in kyphoscoliotic patients (Sinha & Bergofsky 1972), but chest wall and lung compliance in patients with neuromuscular disease did not improve with short term use of IPPB (McCool et al. 1986).

It is unlikely that IPPB provides an advantage in the delivery of drugs over inhalation from a nebulizer by a spontaneously breathing patient. No greater bronchodilator effect was achieved when delivery of a bronchodilator by IPPB was compared to inhalation from a nebulizer in sub-acute asthmatic patients (Webber et al. 1974).

In an exhausted patient with acute severe asthma it may be beneficial to relieve the effort of breathing with IPPB while at the same time delivering bronchodilator drugs. It has been shown that in the completely relaxed subject using IPPB, whether with normal or diseased lungs, the work of breathing during inspiration approaches zero (Ayres et al. 1963).

It has been suggested that IPPB may be of value in patients with chest wall deformity or pronounced inspiratory muscle weakness who cannot voluntarily generate transpulmonary pressures and inspiratory volumes great enough to produce sufficient expiratory flows to aid effective expulsion of secretions (Pontoppidan 1980).

Medical and surgical patients may be exhausted, mentally confused or brain damaged and may be incapable of breathing sufficiently deeply to mobilize bronchial secretions. By using an inspired volume from the IPPB apparatus above the patient's tidal volume, in conjunction with physiotherapy techniques, secretions may be mobilized.

IPPB is not beneficial unless the controls on the apparatus are adjusted carefully to suit the individual, the patient is positioned comfortably to allow relaxation and is given calm and assured instruction by a physiotherapist knowledgeable about the apparatus.

IPPB apparatus

A simple apparatus with minimal controls is most suitable for use with physiotherapy. Two examples of suitable models are the Bird Mark 7 (fig. 84) and Bennett PR–1 (fig. 85). These are pressure-cycled ventilators powered by compressed oxygen or air. Other models, for example, the Bennett AP–5 or Portabird are driven electrically.

The essential features of an IPPB apparatus for use with physiotherapy are:

1 *Positive pressure* range of at least 0–30 cm H_2O.

2 *Simplicity* of controls.

3 *Portability.* The apparatus should be compact and easily movable from patient to patient.

4 *Sensitivity.* The inspiratory phase should be initiated ('triggered') by the patient with minimal effort. Fully automatic control is unpleasant for most patients and unnecessary for physiotherapy, but a hand triggering device is a useful asset.

5 *Flow control.* With machines such as the Bird Mark 7 the inspiratory gas is delivered at a flow rate which can be pre-set by means of a control knob. Optimal distribution of gas is achieved at relatively slow flow rates. However, if the patient is very short of breath and has a fast respiratory rate, a slow inspiratory period may be unacceptable. It will then be necessary to deliver the gas initially at a fast rate. It is important to have the facility for adjusting the flow rate to suit the individual patient.

On the Bennet PR–1 and AP–5 there is

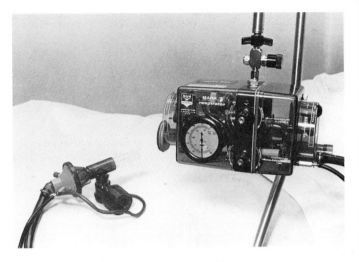

Fig. 84. *Bird Mark 7.*

no adjustment necessary as an automatic variable flow is provided. This is called 'flow sensitivity' and means that the flow of inspired gas adapts to the resistance of the individual patient's airways.

6 *Nebulizer.* An efficient system for nebulization is essential. The machine must never deliver unhumidified gas. If drugs are being administered with the IPPB treatment, the nebulizer must be capable of producing fine particles (p. 131) and of delivering the contents quickly (3–4 ml in 10–15 minutes).

Although the prescribed dosages of bronchodilator drugs may appear large compared to pressurized aerosols, it must be remembered that only 10–20% of the drug reaches the patient, the rest being lost in the equipment and exhaled gas (Shenfield *et al.* 1974).

The Bennett apparatus has a separate control knob for nebulization, but the Bird nebulizer works automatically with the inspiratory phase of the ventilator.

7 *Air-mix control.* If the machine is driven by oxygen it is necessary that air is

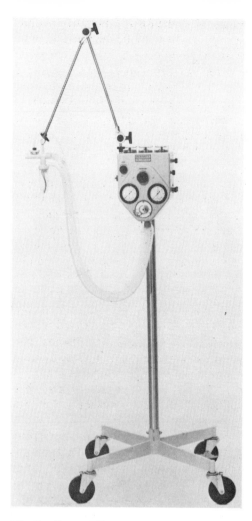

Fig. 85. *Bennett PR–1.*

air with an attachment to provide a controlled, optimal concentration of added oxygen. With the Bird Mark 7, a simple method of achieving a 24% oxygen concentration is to run 2 litres of oxygen through a hypodermic needle into the inlet port of the micro-nebulizer, the machine being driven by compressed air. If a non-compensated oxygen flow meter is used, the flow rate should be set at 2 litres/minute before connecting the tubing in order to obtain an accurate oxygen concentration.

The Bennett PR–1 has a diluter attachment to produce a mixture of air and oxygen.

8 *Mouthpiece or mask.* The majority of patients prefer to use a mouthpiece for IPPB, but a face mask is essential for treatment of confused patients. A silicone rubber flange mouthpiece (fig. 86) is a useful intermediate method for patients who have difficulty making an airtight seal round the mouthpiece.

9 *Breathing-head assembly.* It is most economical to have several sets for each

entrained in order to deliver a mixture of air and oxygen. 100% oxygen should not be delivered to the patient. The Bird Mark 7 is now made without an air-mix control, air being automatically entrained.

Many patients with severe hypoxia require oxygen and it is dangerous to use an IPPB machine delivering air alone (p. 39). If the machine is not powered by oxygen, it can be powered by compressed

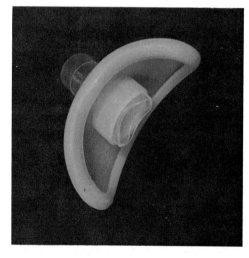

Fig. 86. *Flange mouthpiece (Puritan–Bennett).*

IPPB machine. A breathing-head assembly consists of a mouthpiece or mask, exhalation valve, micro-nebulizer with tubing and two channel tubing which connects the former parts to the machine.

The circuits used will depend on the sterilization policy of the individual hospital. The types available are autoclavable circuits, non-disposable circuits which require non-autoclave sterilization and disposable circuits. To prevent cross infection it is essential for each patient to have a complete breathing-head assembly which is sterilized, or disposed of, at least every week when the course of treatment is completed. The machine itself can be moved from patient to patient.

Preparation for treatment

1 The nebulizer is filled with the required solution. Any drug used in the nebulizer must be prescribed by the physician or surgeon in charge of the patient.

If a bronchodilator is being used in conjunction with the IPPB treatment, the dose of drug is combined with normal saline to give a total of 3 ml of solution. Normal saline solution alone may be used for humidification, but the quantity is unimportant because it is not essential to use up all the solution, or more can be added if required.

2 The breathing-head assembly is connected to the ventilator and the ventilator is connected to the driving gas.

3 The physiotherapist must ensure that the air-mix control is in position for the entrainment of air.

4 If the machine has an expiratory timer (automatic control), this is turned off.

5 The controls of the ventilator are set according to the individual's require-ments. With the Bird Mark 7 the pressure setting is likely to be between 13 and 15 cm H_2O and the flow rate between 6 and 10. The aim is to adjust the pressure and flow controls to provide regular, assisted ventilation without discomfort. A patient with a rigid rib cage will require a higher pressure setting to obtain an adequate tidal gas exchange than someone with a more mobile rib cage. It is sometimes easiest to start with the pressure and flow controls set at 10 and to adjust them as the patient becomes accustomed to using the ventilator. The sensitivity control is usually adjusted to a low figure (5–7) so that minimal inspiratory effort is required. The end of the sensitivity control scale requiring greater effort is only of value when a patient with respiratory muscle weakness is being weaned from a ventilator. Some ventilators have no numbered markings, but having found effective settings for a patient, it is useful to note the position of the controls so that this can be the starting point at the next treatment.

With the Bennett PR–1 the controls to be set are pressure, sensitivity and nebulization.

6 Using the hand triggering device the ventilator is turned on to ensure that the nebulizer is functioning correctly and that there are no leaks in the breathing-head assembly.

Treatment of the patient

The position of the patient depends on the condition for which the IPPB is being given. It may be effectively used in the sitting (fig. 87), high side-lying (fig. 88) or side-lying positions (fig. 89). The patient should be comfortable and able to relax the upper chest and shoulder girdle.

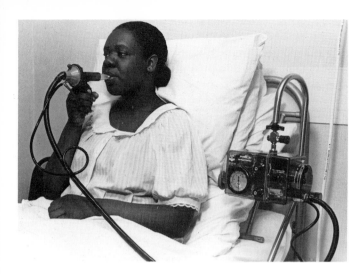

Fig. 87. *IPPB in sitting.*

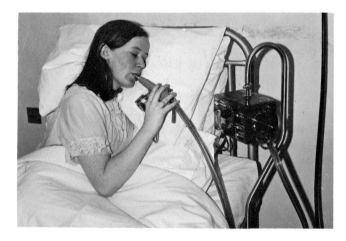

Fig. 88. *IPPB in high side-lying.*

The patient is told to close his lips firmly round the mouthpiece and breathe in through his mouth. After minimal inspiratory effort the machine is triggered into inspiratory flow. The patient should then relax during inspiration, allowing air from the ventilator to inflate his lungs. Provided that he relaxes, the machine will

cycle into expiration when the pre-set pressure is reached at the mouth. If he attempts to assist inspiration, there will be a delay in cycling into expiration. A similar delay occurs if there is any leak around the mouthpiece or mask, or from the patient's nose. It is often necessary to use a nose clip until he becomes accustomed to the ventilator.

Expiration should be quiet and relaxed. Forced expiration with or without IPPB increases the work of breathing and may increase airflow obstruction (p. 16). If the patient exhales before the ventilator cycles into expiration, the needle of the pressure gauge swings round to a higher pressure than that set, while at the same time the machine cycles prematurely into expiration. This too will increase the work of breathing. The movement of the needle is a useful indicator of correct or faulty technique.

The patient relaxes the upper chest and shoulder girdle and the physiotherapist places her hands on the anterior costal margins to encourage gentle movement of the lower chest.

In specific circumstances (p. 127) where expansion is to be emphasized, thoracic expansion exercises may be combined with IPPB, but this will increase the work of breathing.

IPPB, taught correctly, is not exhausting for the patient. The most common faults are the attempt by the patient to assist inspiration either by nose or mouth and premature expiration.

The exhalation valve may be provided with a retard cap which can be used to give resistance to expiration. Unless it is specifically ordered, it is preferable to remove this cap, as it can easily be placed in the wrong position and impede expiration.

To avoid hyperventilation and resultant dizziness, the patient should pause momentarily after expiration, before the next inspiration.

In children it is important to observe the size of the abdomen before, during and after IPPB. Some children tend to swallow air during treatment which may lead to abdominal distension. IPPB should be discontinued if this problem occurs.

Treatment time and frequency of treatment with IPPB depend on the individual case, but it is likely to be between 10 and 20 minutes.

INDICATIONS FOR USE OF IPPB

1 Acute exacerbation of chronic bronchitis

For patients in respiratory failure due to sputum retention, which may occur during an acute exacerbation of chronic bronchitis, treatment with IPPB can be invaluable and intubation frequently avoided (p. 54).

The patient may be confused, drowsy and unable to cough effectively. With this type of patient it is necessary to use the mask and it is helpful to have another physiotherapist or a nurse to assist with the treatment (figs 89 & 90). The patient should be turned on to his side. One physiotherapist, or the nurse, should elevate the jaw and hold the mask firmly over the patient's face ensuring an air-tight fit, whilst the other physiotherapist shakes the chest on expiration. The operator holding the mask may use the manual control on the machine in order to impose effective deep breaths on the patient. After about the first 10 minutes of treatment the patient may become more ratio-

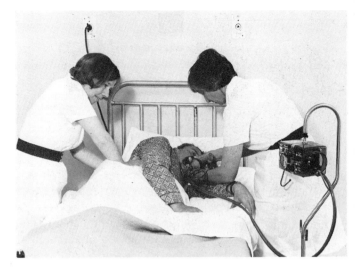

Fig. 89. *IPPB with mask.*

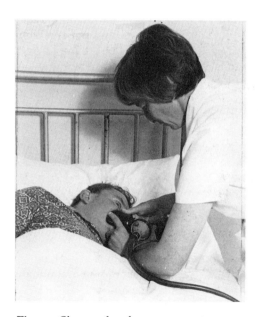

Fig. 90. *Close-up of mask.*

nal and start to cough spontaneously, but if effective coughing is not stimulated, nasopharyngeal suction may be necessary (p. 140).

At first, treatment should be repeated at

125

hourly or 2-hourly intervals. As the patient's condition improves, the frequency of treatment is reduced. It has been shown that a fall in arterial oxygen content can occur as a result of this treatment (Gormezano & Branthwaite 1972b) and therefore each session should be limited to a maximum of 20 minutes.

A bronchodilator drug is usually prescribed to be given in the nebulizer at 4-hourly intervals. Normal saline solution alone is used for the interim treatments.

If any increase in drowsiness is observed while treating the patient, it is probably caused by an increase in arterial carbon dioxide level due to an inadequate tidal gas exchange (Starke et al. 1979). The pressure and flow controls need to be adjusted to increase the tidal volume. With the Bird ventilator an increase in pressure setting will be required and probably an increase in flow rate. A drowsy patient may need encouragement to trigger the machine to maintain an adequate minute ventilation. All patients must be observed for any signs of increased drowsiness during the treatment and for a short period after treatment.

2 Retention of secretions in medical conditions

When tenacious secretions are plugging small airways and cannot be cleared by postural drainage techniques, IPPB may be helpful. This may occur in allergic bronchopulmonary aspergillosis (p. 71) and in some cases of asthma.

If bronchodilator drugs are prescribed these are given by IPPB in a comfortable relaxed position before postural drainage. Physiotherapy and IPPB, using normal saline in the nebulizer, are carried out in

appropriate positions as soon as the bronchodilator has taken effect.

Some patients, with severe bronchiectasis or allergic bronchopulmonary aspergillosis, who have a poor respiratory reserve may benefit from using IPPB during a postural drainage treatment. These patients may be able to do effective breathing techniques, but IPPB may relieve the effort of breathing while mobilizing secretions and after coughing.

3 Acute severe asthma

The majority of asthmatic patients with a severe acute attack respond to bronchodilators inhaled from a simple nebulizer powered by oxygen. A few exhausted asthmatic patients benefit from IPPB which relieves the work of breathing while at the same time delivering the prescribed bronchodilator drugs.

The patient usually finds the high sidelying position (fig. 88) comfortable and may be able to relax his head, shoulders and arms most effectively if the physiotherapist holds the breathing-head assembly for him.

4 Post-operative conditions

Post-operative patients who are too exhausted to carry out effective breathing exercises may benefit from using IPPB or periodic continuous positive airway pressure (PCPAP) to improve ventilation and avoid developing atelectasis.

Normal saline solution is used in the nebulizer, unless a bronchodilator has been prescribed and treatment is given in sitting or any other appropriate position.

Patients who have developed atelectasis or are retaining secretions and are not able to resolve the condition by physiotherapy techniques alone may also benefit from

IPPB or PCPAP. Treatment is given in a postural drainage or modified drainage position. Thoracic expansion exercises may be encouraged during IPPB. In contrast to the usual relaxed technique during the inspiratory phase, inspiration is continued actively to approach total lung capacity. By this means an attempt is being made to increase collateral ventilation and the effect of interdependence (p. 5) to aid re-expansion of the atelectasis.

IPPB is discontinued as soon as the patient is able to breathe deeply enough to mobilize secretions and to huff and cough effectively. IPPB may be required for only 1 or 2 days.

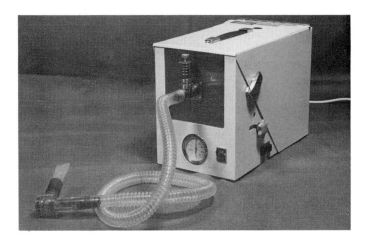

Fig. 91. *Volume cycled IPPB machine—Cape Minor.*

5 Laryngeal dysfunction and phrenic nerve paralysis

Occasionally the larynx is traumatized if an endotracheal tube is in place for several days. If resection of the left recurrent laryngeal nerve is necessary during pneumonectomy, there is difficulty in closure of the vocal cords. In both instances IPPB has been found to be helpful in assisting ventilation and in the removal of secretions.

If the phrenic nerve has been divided during pneumonectomy (p. 92), IPPB may be necessary to assist ventilation post-operatively. The surgeon must give his permission.

6 Chest deformity

Patients with chest wall deformity and respiratory muscle weakness, for example kyphoscoliosis, have a reduced vital capacity. These patients have difficulty clearing excess bronchial secretions during a chest infection and benefit from IPPB used in conjunction with appropriate positioning and physiotherapy. If the rib cage is rigid, a higher pressure setting is required to produce adequate ventilation than for a mobile rib cage.

Long-term domiciliary use of IPPB may be prescribed for kyphoscoliotic patients as it has been shown that lung compliance can be increased by hyper-inflation and the work of breathing decreased (Sinha & Bergofsky 1972). A volume pre-set IPPB device, for example the Cape Minor ventilator (fig. 91), is more effective than a pressure-cycled device in patients with severe restrictive chest wall deformity. The volume pre-set device has produced greater improvement in the patients' vital capacity and this has been maintained for several months (Simonds *et al.* 1986b).

The patient is advised to use the IPPB apparatus for 5 minutes three times daily. The volume is set to give a slight stretch to the chest.

7 Fractured ribs

Patients in road traffic accidents with fractured ribs may have underlying contused lung. If the chest wall is stable, IPPB may help mobilize tenacious blood stained secretions. The possibility of pneumothorax must be eliminated before considering this treatment. Where analgesia is ineffective a localized intercostal nerve block may relieve pain and facilitate more effective physiotherapy.

8 Spinal injuries

The use of IPPB in the acute and non-acute stages of patients with spinal injury is discussed on p. 76.

9 Brain damage

The patient with brain damage may be unable to cooperate with the physiotherapist in maintaining clear airways. IPPB with the face mask to provide periods of effective ventilation, combined with chest vibrations, may be indicated.

10 Weaning from a ventilator

IPPB machines with a sensitivity control can be used in the re-education of paralysed respiratory muscles, for example following acute polyneuritis. The sensitivity control is initially set at a low figure, and then gradually increased to necessitate greater inspiratory effort. In this way the machine may be used to wean patients from non-triggered positive pressure ventilators.

11 Closure of tracheostomy

During the period of healing of a tracheostomy after weaning from a ventilator, the patient may become easily fatigued and unable to clear the airways adequately. IPPB with physiotherapy may assist the patient through this difficult period. For the machine to function correctly, it is often necessary to hold the tracheostomy dressing firmly to prevent any air-leak.

CONTRA-INDICATIONS TO IPPB

1 Pneumothorax

IPPB would tend to increase a pneumothorax and should not be used.

2 Bullae

There is a danger of causing pneumothorax if IPPB is used for a patient with emphysematous bullae.

3 Lung abscess

There is a risk of causing air trapping in the cavity and it is inadvisable to use IPPB for this condition.

4 Haemoptysis

5 Active tuberculosis

6 Cystic fibrosis

Patients with cystic fibrosis have a tendency to pneumothoraces. IPPB should only be used at the request of the physician and the pressure should be kept low. It has also been shown to increase the residual volume in these patients after a prolonged period of treatment (p. 68).

7 Post-operative air leaks

A patient with an intercostal drain to

control an air leak, who also has sputum retention, should only use IPPB with the surgeon's permission. The pressure should be kept low (no higher than 13 cm H_2O).

8 Bronchial tumour in the proximal airways

Air trapping could result if IPPB is used when a tumour is partially obstructing a large bronchus. It could be used to assist clearance of bronchial secretions if the tumour is in the peripheral airways.

Sterilization of equipment

Each patient should have his own breathing-head assembly to minimize the risks of cross infection.

After each treatment the mouthpiece is scrubbed with warm water and the nebulizer is rinsed and dried. The tubing is detached from the ventilator and the complete assembly stored in a polythene bag or other suitable container until required again. After the course of treatment the entire breathing-head assembly is sterilized unless it is a disposable item.

A ventilator used for a patient with particularly resistant strains of bacteria should be confined to that patient and it should be sterilized before use with another patient. The ventilator may be sterilized with ethylene oxide gas.

Servicing of equipment

The IPPB machine should be cleaned internally and overhauled at least every 12 months.

It is important to keep a stock of spare parts so that any perishable or breakable parts can be replaced quickly.

PERIODIC CONTINUOUS POSITIVE AIRWAY PRESSURE (PCPAP)

Periodic continuous positive airway pressure (PCPAP) is the periodic application of a positive airway pressure throughout inspiration and expiration during spontaneous breathing.

Continuous positive airway pressure (CPAP) has been used in the medical world for over 50 years (Poulton 1936), but PCPAP has been used by physiotherapists as a mechanical adjunct only in recent years (Renwick 1985).

A high flow generator is required to provide and to maintain flow rates which will greatly exceed the patient's inspiratory demand. PCPAP can be administered via a mask or a mouthpiece with a nose clip (fig. 92).

The effects of PCPAP are an increase in functional residual capacity and a reduction in the work of breathing (Gherini et al. 1979). PCPAP may increase the collateral ventilation (p. 4) of poorly ventilated or non-ventilated air spaces and aid re-expansion of atelectatic areas by this mechanism. It has been shown to be an effective means of administering bronchodilator drugs (Andersen & Klausen 1982) and has been used in the treatment of atelectasis (Andersen et al. 1980).

The proximal airway pressure during PCPAP must be maintained at a constant level throughout the respiratory cycle. If it drops during inspiration, added inspiratory work will be imposed and if it rises above the set level during expiration, added expiratory work is required. The

129

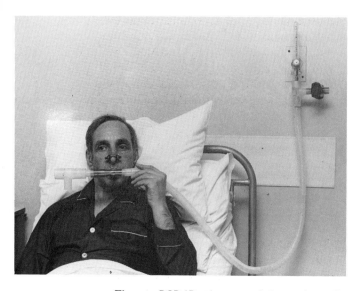

Fig. 92. *PCPAP using a mouthpiece and noseclip (Medic-Aid).*

intrapleural and intrapulmonary changes are similar to the changes occurring during spontaneous breathing. The mechanical work of breathing is reduced owing to the increase in lung compliance.

The uses of PCPAP are:
1 Re-expansion of atelectasis.
2 Prevention of atelectasis.
3 Reduction in the work of breathing.
4 Mobilization of excess bronchial secretions.

The contra-indications are the same as for IPPB (p. 128). In children it is important to observe the size of the abdomen before, during and after PCPAP. Some children may swallow air during treatment which may lead to abdominal distension. PCPAP should be discontinued if this problem occurs.

Technique of treatment

The patient is comfortably positioned, either in the sitting position or in the drainage position for the affected lung segment or lung (fig. 93). The PCPAP is given for 2–4 minutes while the patient relaxes his upper chest and shoulders and is encouraged to breathe gently with his lower chest. A valve giving a positive end expiratory pressure (PEEP) of 5, 7·5 or 10 cmH$_2$O is usually suitable.

The period of CPAP is followed by the use of the forced expiration technique (p. 21) and this cycle is repeated for 15 to 20 minutes. The treatment session is repeated as necessary. Chest clapping and shaking with PCPAP may negate some of the effect of the CPAP if these manoeuvres reduce functional residual capacity (Falk *et al.* 1984).

Care must be taken when a fixed inspiratory oxygen flow generator is used in the treatment of patients with hypercapnia. An adjustable inspiratory oxygen flow generator is available or the fixed flow generator can be run from an air supply.

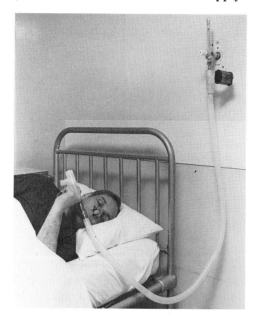

Fig. 93. *PCPAP in side-lying.*

A nebulizer with a prescribed broncho-dilator may be included in the circuit. Humidification is provided by the air entrained by the device. Additional humidification may be included in the circuit, but is usually unnecessary for the short periods of treatment.

Further clinical studies are needed, but PCPAP appears to be a simple and useful mechanical adjunct in clinical practice.

NEBULIZATION

A nebulizer is a means of administering drugs by inhalation. It breaks up the solution to be inhaled into fine droplets which are then suspended in a stream of gas. The patient actively inhales this gas stream containing the drug.

The deposition of droplets within the respiratory tract is dependent partly on the size of the droplets produced by the nebulizer. In the upper airways where the total cross-sectional diameter of the airway is small and the airflow high, droplets deposit by inertial impaction on the airway walls as the airstream changes direction. Droplets depositing by impaction are in the range 5–10 μm.

Beyond the 10th generation of bronchi the total cross-sectional area of the airway increases rapidly and there is a significant slowing of airflow. Droplets of 0.5–5 μm deposit in the small airways and alveoli by gravitational sedimentation as a result of the low flow, those less than 2 μm reaching the alveoli.

The aerosol coming from a nebulizer usually contains droplets of many different sizes and the output characteristic for an individual nebulizer is best described by the mass median aerodynamic diameter (MMAD). Half of the aerosol mass is contained in droplets smaller than the MMAD and half of the aerosol mass in droplets larger than the MMAD. The ideal size for a therapeutic aerosol is not known, but the MMAD should be no greater than 5 μm if peripheral deposition is required (Newman & Clarke 1983). A recent study suggests that a nebulizer giving droplets with the MMAD less than 2 μm should be used to maximize lung deposition (Clay & Clarke 1987), but Mitchell et al. (1987) show no difference in bronchodilator effect comparing aerosols of 1·4 μm and 5·5 μm MMAD.

The pattern of deposition within the bronchial tree depends not only on droplet size, but also on the method of inhalation and on the degree of airflow obstruction (Newman et al. 1986). Rapid inhalation increases deposition in the large airways, while slow deep inhalation probably results in more peripheral deposition. In patients with airflow obstruction the droplets tend to deposit more centrally because of narrowing of the airways with bronchospasm or excess secretions.

The patient should be in a well-supported position and with the upper chest relaxed should attempt to breathe slowly and deeply using the lower chest. After about three deep breaths he should breathe gently using the lower chest (breathing control). If encouraged to breathe deeply throughout the entire nebulizer treatment the patient would suffer from the effects of hyperventilation. This technique of alternating deep breaths with breathing control may provide better distribution of the nebulized droplets than breathing at tidal volume throughout. The potential use of breath holding during nebulization is under investigation.

A face mask is less efficient than a

mouthpiece as a means of delivering nebulized drugs. It has been shown that using a mask much of the drug is deposited on the face and in the upper respiratory tract (Wolfsdorf *et al.* 1969). A mouthpiece is attached to the nebulizer with an aperture in the system for entrainment of air during inspiration and for exhalation. The patient is then able to keep his mouth closed round the mouthpiece throughout the inhalation treatment. It may be necessary to remind the patient to remove the mouthpiece momentarily to swallow, if saliva collects in the mouth. If the saliva should be dribbled into the nebulizer, treatment time is unnecessarily prolonged.

In addition to less effective deposition of the inhaled drug when using a face mask, a further disadvantage is the drug being deposited in the nose, on the skin and in the eyes. Inhaled antibiotics and corticosteroids should not be allowed on the face and Atrovent should not enter the eyes. It may be necessary to use a face mask for a small child, but this should be replaced by a mouthpiece as soon as he can manage.

An ideal nebulizer should be efficient, simple, reliable, easy to clean, inexpensive and capable of producing droplets with the MMAD of no more than 5 μm. There are two types of nebulizer in clinical use, the jet nebulizer and ultrasonic nebulizer.

Jet nebulizers

There are many models available, but they work on a similar principle. A high velocity jet of gas is blown through a fine hole creating an area of negative pressure. Fluid is drawn from the reservoir by the Bernouilli effect into the jet stream and is impacted on a baffle breaking the fluid into droplets. Large droplets fall back into the reservoir while the smaller ones may be inhaled.

The rate at which the drug is delivered from the jet nebulizer and the size of the droplets depend not only on the construction of the nebulizer, but also on the power of the driving source. A larger proportion of small droplets are produced if the flow rate is 6–8 litres/minute in preference to 4 litres/minute (Clay *et al.* 1983).

In hospital it is often convenient to power a nebulizer with 6–8 litres/minute from the piped oxygen supply and in hypoxic patients without carbon dioxide retention it is important to use oxygen. For those patients with a raised carbon dioxide level who are dependent on this hypoxic drive to stimulate breathing the nebulizer should be powered from an air source (Gunawardena *et al.* 1984). Piped air may not be available and an air compressor is often more convenient than using air cylinders in hospital.

An air compressor for inhalation treatment should be oil-free, portable, durable, as quiet as possible and capable of producing an adequate pressure and flow of air. Bronchodilator drugs require a compressor producing a flow of 6–8 litres/minute, but the viscous antibiotic drugs need a compressor with a flow of at least 9 litres/minute in order that the treatment time is not excessive.

With all jet nebulizers there is a volume of solution (approximately 1 ml) left in the nebulizer after it has run to 'dryness'. The patient is encouraged to tap the side of the nebulizer to allow as much as possible to be delivered, but it should be explained that there is always some residue. It is important to use a minimum of 3 ml of solution and preferably 4 ml in order to deliver an adequate percentage of the prescribed drug. In an assessment of jet nebulizers when 2 ml was used, only 50% of the dose was released as aerosol, whereas with a volume of 4 ml 60–80% was released (Clay *et al.* 1983).

Ultrasonic nebulizers

High frequency sound waves are passed through a solution in a reservoir to create an aerosol. Ultrasonic nebulizers for delivery of small quantities of drug are used less often than jet nebulizers in Britain. An advantage of ultrasonic nebulizers is that they operate quietly but they are less robust and need more careful maintenance than jet nebulizers and air compressors.

Some of these nebulizers are dependent on the patient's ability to breathe in actively to open a valve. Some children and other patients with poor lung function may find this difficult.

If antibiotics are inhaled from one of these nebulizers, a one-way valve system must be fitted to vent the exhaled antibiotic.

INDICATIONS FOR THE USE OF NEBULIZERS

1 Delivery of bronchodilator drugs

Bronchodilator drugs can be delivered to patients who are shown to have a greater response to the nebulized drug than to the other forms of administration (p. 43). In an acute attack of asthma (p. 57) a nebulizer is the most common means of delivery. Respiratory patients who are too short of breath to use a pressurized aerosol or rotahaler effectively may be prescribed nebulized bronchodilators if some reversibility of the airways is anticipated.

2 Infants and children with asthma

Inhalation by nebulizer is the only means of effective inhalation therapy until a child is about 4 years old (p. 59). Bronchodilator drugs and sodium cromoglycate (Intal) can be inhaled by this method. Beclomethasone diproprionate is available as a nebulizer suspension, but it may not be as effective as other methods of administering corticosteroids (Reiser & Warner 1986).

3 Administration of antibiotics and antifungal agents

In some cases of resistant chest infections, for example in cystic fibrosis (p. 67) or bronchiectasis, antibiotics may be prescribed to be inhaled directly into the lungs. The nebulizer should be fitted with a one-way valve system and wide bore tubing (fig. 94) to allow the exhaled gas to

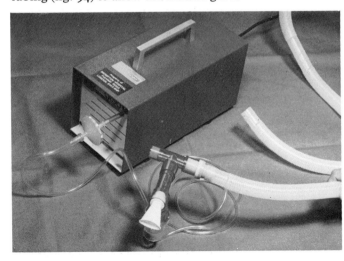

Fig. 94. *Compressor, nebulizer and 1-way valve system for inhalation of antibiotics (Medic-Aid CR60 and System 22).*

133

be vented out through a window. This is necessary to prevent small quantities of antibiotics remaining in the atmosphere with the result that dormant organisms may become resistant to the antibiotics. A nose clip is necessary if the patient is breathing partially through his nose. It is important to use a powerful air compressor, giving a flow of at least 9 litres/minute, when nebulizing the more viscous antibiotics.

When two antibiotics are to be inhaled it is usually necessary to inhale them separately. Mixing them in the nebulizer can cause inactivation of some drugs. If a 2 ml dose of an antibiotic is prescribed, it is necessary to add 1–2 ml of the appropriate diluent (normal saline or sterile water) to make the total solution up to an adequate volume (p. 132). The pharmacist should be consulted about the correct solutions for dilution and the advisability of mixing drugs.

Antifungal drugs, such as natamycin (Pimafucin) or Brilliant Green, are sometimes inhaled in the treatment of aspergilloma or bronchopulmonary aspergillosis. In all these cases if postural drainage is carried out, it should precede the inhalation.

4 Aid to expectoration

Some physicians prescribe mucolytic drugs, while others feel that normal saline solution delivered as a mist may be equally effective. Inhalation of hypertonic (7%) saline has been found to increase clearance of bronchial secretions in some patients (Pavia et al. 1978). Patients with cystic fibrosis occasionally find it helpful to inhale hypertonic saline before postural drainage. In a few patients it may cause an increase in airflow obstruction (Schoeffel

et al. 1981). Assessment using peak expiratory flow or vitalograph recordings before and after the first inhalation is advisable.

Inhalation of hypertonic saline may assist production of sputum for diagnostic purposes when the patient has failed to produce any sputum with physiotherapy alone.

Acetylcysteine is occasionally prescribed, but may have an irritant effect producing hypersecretion and may reduce the viscosity of the secretions to the extent that they are difficult to expectorate. Changes in airflow obstruction should be assessed at the first treatment. A nebulizer delivering acetylcysteine should be driven by an air supply because oxygen inactivates the drug.

5 Local analgesia

Inhalation of Marcain (3–4 ml of 0·5% Marcain plain) may be useful in patients with intractable cough which may occur with fibrosing alveolitis, or viral infections affecting the irritant or cough receptors in the mucosa of the large airways. A study has shown that the period of freedom from persistent cough may last up to 6 weeks (Howard et al. 1977). It is presumed that a reflex cycle is broken to produce this prolonged response to the drug. Treatment is repeated according to the individual's symptoms and in some cases is required as often as three times a day. It is advisable that the patient does not eat or drink for an hour and a half after the inhalation. Marcain is used in preference to Lignocaine as the analgesic effect is of longer duration and it also has a more favourable therapeutic/toxic ratio.

It has also been suggested that suppression of the J-receptors in the alveoli may relieve dyspnoea in patients with the intractable dyspnoea of severe fibrosing alveolitis, or in some terminally ill patients such as those suffering from alveolar carcinoma. Marcain has been used in an attempt to suppress the J-receptors, but no formal trial has yet been completed.

DOMICILIARY USE OF NEBULIZERS

Indications

Patients requiring domiciliary equipment should be carefully selected and only those benefiting from treatment that cannot be given in any simpler form should be loaned equipment.

A few severe asthmatic patients who have life-threatening falls in peak expiratory flow rate in the night or early morning, may respond better to nebulized bronchodilator drugs than to other methods of inhalation during these acute episodes. Other asthmatic patients may require a trial period at home recording objective information on a diary card. A peak flow chart can be used before and after inhalation of bronchodilator drugs. Provided that other drug therapy is not changed during the period, a trial for 1 month of simple bronchodilator inhalation (pressurized aerosol or rotahaler) may be compared to 1 month using nebulized bronchodilators. Young children with asthma may require a nebulizer until they are old enough to manage the simpler devices (p. 59).

Patients with chronic airflow obstruction often feel subjective benefit from nebulized bronchodilator drugs, but should have a trial using spirometry recording FEV_1 and FVC to determine whether greater benefit is gained from the nebulizer than from the simpler forms of delivery (p. 43).

Patients requiring inhaled antibiotics or antifungal drugs need domiciliary equipment. Cystic fibrosis patients often need inhalations from a nebulizer before and after postural drainage (p. 67).

Disadvantages

Equipment and drugs for nebulization are expensive and should not be provided unless necessary. Some patients respond adequately to bronchodilator drugs by pressurized aerosol or rotahaler during the day time, but may benefit from a nebulizer at night and in the early morning. It is important that they do not become unnecessarily dependent on the nebulizer for all doses of bronchodilators because this may limit their life style.

There is a possible danger of a patient overusing bronchodilator drugs when other drug treatment is indicated. It is essential that instruction is given by the doctor and reinforced by the physiotherapist, that the patient must not place too much reliance on the nebulizer. If it is not having its usual effect, the patient should seek medical advice.

Equipment

An electric air compressor and nebulizer system should be supplied that is suited to the drugs required and the patient's circumstances. Inhaled antibiotics need a more powerful compressor (fig. 94, p. 133) than bronchodilator drugs (fig. 95). Patients who may need to use a nebulizer while travelling by car should

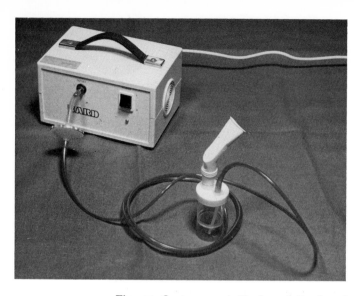

Fig. 95. *Compressor suitable for nebulization of bronchodilator drugs (Bard).*

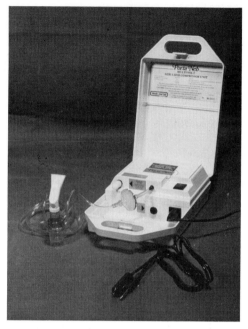

Fig. 96. *Compressor with an adaptor for operation from a battery (Portaneb Multivolt, Medic-Aid).*

have a system that can function from a car battery (fig. 96).

A patient who travels abroad should be advised to take an international travel plug adaptor and if he is visiting a country using a different electric voltage, a transformer or dual voltage compressor is required. A letter from a doctor to show to the Customs officials is a sensible precaution to explain the reason for travelling with drugs and possibly syringes and needles.

A foot pump to power a nebulizer is obtainable, but requires considerable energy to operate. It can be useful in circumstances where no electricity is available.

The standard British domiciliary flow head fitted to an oxygen cylinder is unsuitable as the driving source for a nebulizer as it has a maximum output of only 4 litres/minute. A flow meter permitting higher flows of oxygen could be used,

but is expensive and more restricting to the patient's lifestyle than a portable compressor.

Patient instruction

Careful instruction must be given to the patient in the technique of inhaling from a nebulizer and in the use and care of the equipment. He must be supervised in filling the nebulizer with the prescribed drugs. The nebulizer must be rinsed after each treatment to keep the jets clear and it should be sterilized at home weekly with Milton solution.

The patient should always have a spare nebulizer available and a spare air inlet filter. Arrangements must be made for regular annual servicing of air compressors and emergency servicing if necessary.

HUMIDIFICATION

During normal respirations the inspired air is warmed and humidified by the mucus membranes, so that it is fully saturated at body temperature when it reaches the trachea. If with disease there is fever, hyperventilation or dehydration, the mucosa of the upper airways may become dehydrated. If there is not sufficient moisture available to replace that used up in humidifying the inspired air, cilial activity is decreased, because efficient action of the cilia is dependent on continuous moistening of the respiratory mucosa (p. 4). Dehydration also makes bronchial secretions become thick and viscid. The combination of these tenacious secretions with depressed cilial activity makes expectoration difficult.

Distressed breathless patients often do not drink enough and if fluids are given by mouth or infusion, the secretions will become less tenacious. Humidification of the inspired air or oxygen may also assist in loosening secretions and aid expectoration.

Humidity can be obtained in two different ways, either by inhaling water vapour or inhaling a mist of nebulized particles.

The first method is the principle of the hot water humidifier where gas is blown over the heated water and it absorbs water vapour which is then inhaled by the patient.

Nebulizers produce a mist of particles which are suspended in a stream of gas and then inhaled. Small nebulizers with a high output (p. 132) can be used for humidification, but large volume jet nebulizers are often more convenient. Some jet nebulizers can have a heater incorporated in the system to provide a stream of heated mist for inhalation. Many patients with airflow obstruction react adversely to inhalation of a cold vapour and to hypotonic or hypertonic solutions (Schoeffel 1981). Careful assessment is necessary and a more favourable response is likely to heated humidity compared with cold humidity.

Ultrasonic nebulizers produce a dense mist of very fine particles which may possibly be inhaled further into the respiratory tract than those producing larger particles. Many ultrasonic nebulizers do not have a heater, but the temperature of the mist is not as cold as that from a nebulizer powered from a piped oxygen supply.

Devices which bubble the inspired gas through cold water are not an effective means of humidification, but are useful for patients requiring oxygen by nasal cannulae to prevent uncomfortable drying of the nasal mucosa.

Regular sterilization of all humidifiers is essential to prevent infection.

INDICATIONS FOR HUMIDIFICATION

1 Humidification with controlled oxygen therapy

Many patients who require controlled oxygen therapy, such as a chronic bronchitic with an acute exacerbation, have viscid tenacious secretions. Controlled oxygen is often provided by means of a Ventimask connected to the oxygen supply by a narrow bore tube. Effective humidification via narrow bore tubing is impossible due to condensation.

A device known as a humidity adapter can be used, whereby the air entrained by the mask is humidified. It is a cuff which partially surrounds the air entraining holes of the Ventimask (fig. 97) and is connected by wide bore tubing to a humidifier. The humidifier must be powered by an air source. This can be piped air if it is available, an air cylinder or an electric air compressor capable of continuous use (figs 98 & 99). An ultrasonic nebulizer, set at a high flow, can be used and has the advantage of being quieter than a jet nebulizer system.

2 Tenacious secretions in medical chest disease

Inhalations of normal saline (0·9%) or sterile water by mouthpiece, for 10–15 minutes preceding postural drainage are helpful in exacerbations of cystic fibrosis (p. 67), in allergic bronchopul-

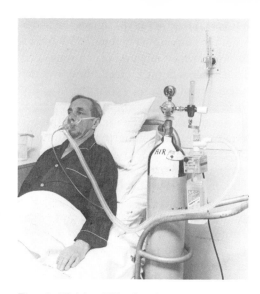

Fig. 98. *High humidification of 24% oxygen, with an air cylinder.*

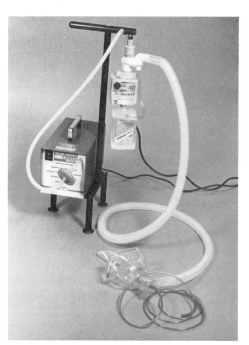

Fig. 97. *Ventimask with humidity adaptor and humidification system (Vickers, Medic-Aid, Kendall).*

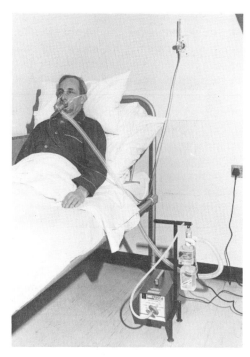

Fig. 99. *High humidification of 24% oxygen with an air compressor.*

monary aspergillosis (p. 71) and in occasional cases of asthma with severe plugging of the airways. Humidifiers particularly successful with these conditions are ultrasonic nebulizers (fig. 100), or nebulizers incorporating a heating device.

Treatment can be repeated 2 hourly if necessary. It is important to test the patient's FEV₁ or PEFR before and after inhaling from the humidifier, to ensure that no deterioration has been caused. The recordings after inhalation should not be taken immediately following a bout of coughing. A true reading should be obtained after the airways have had a short period to relax.

3 Post-operative sputum retention

If a patient is wearing a mask giving an oxygen concentration of 28% or more, one of the large volume nebulizers with high density output can be connected by wide bore tubing to the mask to provide effective humidification.

Intermittent inhalations by mouth (fig. 101) are often helpful preceding breathing exercises and huffing or postural drainage. Simple steam inhalations can be useful provided the patient inspires deeply and precautions are taken to avoid spillage.

4 Infants and children

The narrow airways in childhood make the provision of high humidification particularly important, both when the child is intubated and non-intubated. This is discussed in Chapter 10 (p. 150).

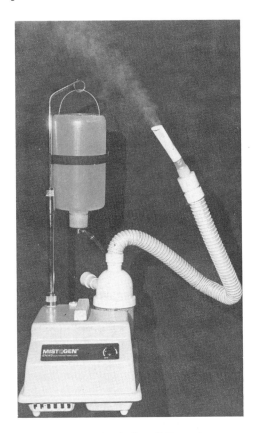

Fig. 100. *Ultrasonic nebulizer (Mistogen).*

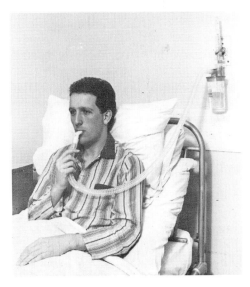

Fig. 101. *Humidification from a large volume nebulizer (Misty Ox, Medic-Acid).*

5 Intubated patients

A hot water humidifier may be incorporated into the respiratory circuit of an intubated adult patient, but a vapour condenser humidifier is usually a satisfactory alternative and avoids the potential risk of infection of water humidifiers.

The condenser humidifier is a lightweight disposable device fitted on to the endotracheal tube swivel connection. It contains a material which is an efficient heat and moisture exchanger. This material picks up the warmth and moisture of the exhaled air as it passes through to the atmosphere and during inspiration the air absorbs the warmth and moisture on its way to the lungs. The humidifier is changed every 24 hours or immediately if it becomes soiled with secretions.

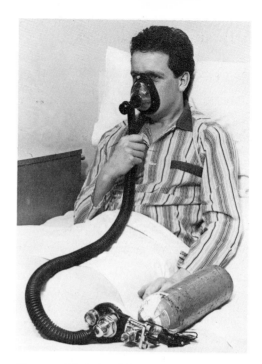

Fig. 102. *Inhalation of Entonox (BOC).*

ENTONOX

Entonox is pre-mixed oxygen (50%) and nitrous oxide (50%) and is an analgesic which may be administered using a patient-demand valve (Myles 1970) and a mask or mouthpiece (fig. 102). Entonox provides rapid onset analgesia, but its effect lasts only as long as the gas is inhaled (Seal 1974).

The *uses* of Entonox are in the treatment of patients with acute or chronic chest pain, for example steroid induced rib fracture and post-operative pain inhibiting effective huffing and coughing. The *contra-indications* are pre-existing nausea, gaseous abdominal distension, pneumothorax and lung abscess. The gas will diffuse into air pockets and increase their volume. The most common *side effect* is a tendency to feel sleepy and this can be avoided if the patient is allowed to hold

the mask or mouthpiece in position. Euphoria is often experienced.

NASOPHARYNGEAL SUCTION IN ADULTS

Nasopharyngeal suction, as a means of stimulating a cough, is an unpleasant procedure for the patient and should be performed only when absolutely necessary. The indication for suction is the inability to cough effectively and expectorate when secretions are being retained. It may be necessary in such conditions as respiratory failure due to acute exacerbations of chronic bronchitis (p. 125), post-operative complications, laryngeal dysfunction or neurological disorders.

It is contra-indicated when there is severe bronchospasm or stridor.

Technique

This procedure is carried out through the nose in adults. A soft catheter of suitable size should be lubricated with a water soluble jelly, and gently passed through the nasal passage so that it curves down into the pharynx. Effective coughing is often stimulated with the catheter in this position. Suction should not be connected until the catheter is in the pharynx.

In adults it may be possible to pass the catheter between the vocal cords and into the trachea. If the patient is able to cooperate this is easier to perform if the neck is extended and with the tongue protruding. The catheter should be inserted during the inspiratory phase and if it is passed into the trachea, vigorous coughing will be stimulated.

It is important to observe the patient for signs of anoxia during the procedure and oxygen should be available.

If it has been difficult to insert the catheter and the patient looks cyanosed, instead of withdrawing the catheter, the suction should be disconnected and oxygen administered until the patient's colour has improved, then suction should be reconnected.

Adults who are nursed sitting up in bed, can be suctioned in that position, whereas comatose patients are usually suctioned while lying on their side.

Nasopharyngeal suction is contra-indicated in patients with head injuries where there is a leak of cerebrospinal fluid into the nasal passages. Oropharyngeal suction through an airway is used as an alternative method.

Some authorities feel that the technique of passing the catheter into the trachea should not be used because of the risks of causing laryngeal spasm or vagal stimulation (Sykes *et al.* 1976). However, others find that it is a valuable technique provided it is carried out carefully and oxygen is always available.

Nasopharyngeal suction is a procedure that should not be undertaken until every attempt to achieve effective coughing has failed. Alternative treatments available would be minitracheotomy, bronchoscopy or temporary intubation, but these can very often be avoided by the use of careful suction.

MINITRACHEOTOMY

There are occasions when a patient retains bronchial secretions and could develop respiratory failure despite active efforts of the physiotherapist. Nasopharyngeal/tracheal suction may have been successful in clearing secretions, but if it is necessary to repeat this frequently it is unpleasant and traumatic for the patient.

In these circumstances a minitracheotomy is a means of clearing secretions easily and avoiding the more invasive techniques of bronchoscopy, endotracheal intubation or tracheostomy.

A cannula with an internal diameter of 4 mm is inserted into the trachea through the cricothyroid membrane (Matthews & Hopkinson 1984). It can be inserted under local anaesthesia and when it is in place tracheal suction can be carried out, as frequently as necessary, using a 10 FG suction catheter. The tube is held in position by tapes around the patient's neck and a spigot is fitted in the opening of the tube except during suction (fig. 103).

The small tracheal tube allows the

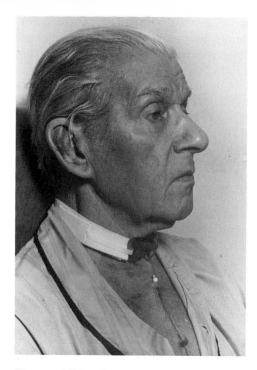

Fig. 103. *Minitracheotomy.*

patient to breathe normally through the mouth and nose. He is humidifying the air passing through the nasal passages and does not usually require additional humidification. Important advantages of minitracheotomy over other forms of intubation are that the patient can talk, eat and drink normally and the tube does not prevent him from coughing effectively. If a patient requires oxygen it is given by a face mask or nasal cannulae. These are humidified by the usual methods (p. 137).

Suction is carried out with sterile technique. The small bore of the minitracheotomy will allow the patient to breathe during the procedure. A size 10 FG catheter is the maximum size that can be used, size 8 FG is usually too narrow to clear secretions effectively. 1–2 ml of normal saline solution is instilled via the tube before suction. The catheter is gently inserted and suction is applied when withdrawal of the catheter begins. There are often copious secretions which take longer to clear with this small catheter, but because the patient can continue breathing with the narrow-sized tracheal tube *in situ* he is not distressed by the procedure.

Breathing exercises, breathing control and the forced expiration technique are carried out by the physiotherapist in positions appropriate for the individual patient. He is encouraged to huff and cough with suction being used as necessary.

The minitracheotomy is removed when the patient is capable of clearing his secretions effectively without becoming exhausted. The small incision heals quickly and is often airtight within 1 day.

The minitracheotomy was designed for the adult trachea, the size being adequate both for normal breathing around the tube and suction from within. The minitracheotomy is not recommended for children under the age of 12 years (Preston *et al.* 1986).

Minitracheotomy has been successfully used in surgical and medical patients (Preston *et al.* 1986) and is of great benefit in avoiding a respiratory crisis.

GLOSSOPHARYNGEAL BREATHING

Glossopharyngeal breathing (GPB) is a useful method of independent breathing and assisted coughing in patients with paralysis of the respiratory muscles. It was first described by Dail (1951) when patients with poliomyelitis were observed to be gulping air into their lungs. The name 'frog breathing' is often used, because of the similarity to the breathing mechanism of amphibians.

GPB is a form of positive pressure breathing produced by the patient's voluntary muscles instead of a mechanical ventilator. Some patients with poliomyelitis who have been entirely dependent on a mechanical ventilator for respiration are able to use GPB continuously during their waking hours as a substitute for the mechanical device. Many paralysed patients who have sufficient muscle power to breathe independently of a ventilator have a reduced vital capacity and an inadequate cough. An important use of GPB is to produce an effective cough in these patients. It can also help them to shout if they need to attract attention and it may assist in maintaining or improving compliance of the lungs and chest wall.

During inspiration a series of pumping strokes is performed by action of the lips, mouth, tongue, soft palate, pharynx and larynx. The larynx acts as an intermittent valve to hold the air in the chest. Expiration is passive.

Individual techniques vary, but each pumping stroke takes about 0·6 seconds (Dail *et al.* 1955) and is repeated rapidly until the required volume of air is obtained. If it is being used continuously, in place of tidal breathing, about 6–8 gulps may be taken before exhaling. If it is being used to obtain a maximal vital capacity to produce an effective cough, between 10–20 gulps may be required depending on the stroke volume of each gulp. In a study by Kelleher & Parida (1957) the average volume of each gulp for individual patients varied between 25 ml and 120 ml. When teaching GPB an attempt should be made to reach a volume of at least 60 ml per gulp.

Teaching GPB

Some patients learn GPB easily, but others need time and patience to acquire the technique and must be prepared to practise frequently during the learning phase. It is easier to learn by watching someone adept at the technique than by studying the written word.

A preliminary step to obtain the feeling of holding air in the chest is to use a volume cycled IPPB machine (fig. 91, p. 127) with a mouthpiece. A technique of 'summation' is useful where one breath is held in the chest and a second breath is added so that the patient feels the stretch of his lungs and prevents escape of air through the larynx or nose between the two breaths.

The next and most important step is to gain up-and-down movement of the cartilages while keeping the jaw still. The patient can feel movement of the Adam's apple with his fingers and watch the movement in a mirror.

Having achieved this movement, progression is made to a cycle of three steps, practised slowly at first:
(a) The mouth is opened, the Adam's apple depressed, the jaw remains still and the base of the tongue is depressed keeping the tip against the lower teeth. This step makes space for air in the mouth and pharynx (fig. 104).
(b) Maintaining the position obtained in step (a), the lips are closed trapping the air (fig. 105).
(c) The floor of the mouth is relaxed as the Adam's apple is allowed to rise back into its normal position. During this phase

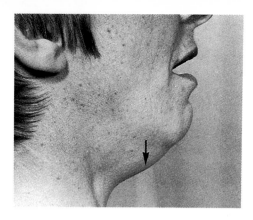

Fig. 104. *GPB step a.*

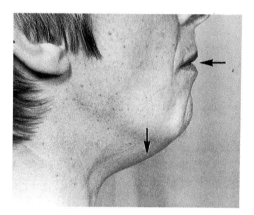

Fig. 105. *GPB step b.*

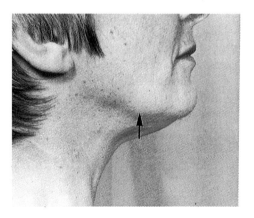

Fig. 106. *GPB step c.*

the air is pumped through the opened larynx into the trachea (fig. 106).

These three movements can be gradually speeded up, until the cycle becomes a flowing movement. At first, air may escape via the nose during step (c) and a nose clip may be required until the soft palate prevents this leak of air.

The patient then takes his maximum breath in, holds it and immediately gulps air by GPB to augment his vital capacity. Using a Wright's respirometer with a mouthpiece on the expiratory limb, the physiotherapist can discover if the patient is achieving GPB. This technique can be used to try and improve the gulp volume, attempting to increase the augmented vital capacity with less gulps.

Having achieved the technique in a comfortable sitting position, it should be practised in positions useful for assisted coughing. The patient fills his chest to capacity, gives the physiotherapist a signal and compression of the chest is applied as the patient lets the air out of his chest. Some patients can apply compression with their own arms, others will need assistance from relatives or friends. The techniques can be used in conjunction with postural drainage if the patient has excess bronchial secretions.

Indications and contra-indications

Teaching GPB should be considered when treating tetraplegic or poliomyelitis patients with a reduced vital capacity (less than 2 litres) and ineffective cough. Instruction should not be started in the acute phase of the condition nor when the patient has an acute chest infection, but should begin as soon as a stable stage is reached and the patient is prepared to practise. Having learnt the technique it can be used with good effect during an acute chest infection (p. 77).

Patients with neuromuscular disorders affecting swallowing should not attempt to learn the technique and it may be unsuitable for those who have a progressive neuromuscular disorder. IPPB is an easier alternative to assist in overcoming chest infections and to maintain compliance in these patients. GPB is contraindicated in patients with pulmonary disease and airflow obstruction.

DEVELOPMENT OF THE RESPIRATORY SYSTEM IN THE INFANT

There are several anatomical and physiological differences in infants, compared with the older child and adult, which lead to different respiratory problems and treatment requirements.

By the 16th week of gestation all the conducting airways have developed and they gradually increase in length and calibre as the child grows. Cartilage develops in the airways from the 24th week of gestation and smooth muscle fibres are present in the airway walls during the last few weeks of gestation, but do not become abundant until the infant is several months old. Goblet cells and mucus glands are well developed at birth (Escobedo 1982).

Progressive development of primitive alveoli occurs from the 16th to 40th week of gestation. At term only 8% of the total adult number of alveoli are present. Further development consists of a combination of multiplication of alveoli and an increase in their size until approximately the 8th year of age. The latter continues until the chest wall stops growing (Pang & Mellins 1975). Collateral ventilation is not fully developed in infancy and is a factor predisposing to atelectasis.

The terminal airspaces are lined with two types of cells. Type I are flat cells responsible for gas exchange and type II cells produce surfactant, a phospholipid, which is delivered to the alveolar surface forming a film which lowers its surface tension. Surfactant is present in the type II cells between 26 and 28 weeks' gestation, but it is not delivered to the epithelial surface until about the 30th week. Without surfactant, small alveoli empty into the larger alveoli and atelectasis develops.

In infancy the rib cage is floppy and compliant. The ribs are horizontally placed and the sternum is softer than that of an adult. The normal breathing pattern is abdominal movement rather than rib cage movement. The 'bucket-handle' movement of the ribs is absent because of the horizontal positioning of the ribs and the poorly developed intercostal muscles. The diaphragm, which is largely responsible for inspiration, is flatter than in the adult. The angle of insertion of the adult diaphragm is oblique, whereas it inserts almost horizontally in the neonate (Muller & Bryan 1979). It is therefore working at a mechanical disadvantage in the infant.

The intercostal muscles are required to act as fixators to support the compliant rib cage and the abdominal muscles work to stabilize the abdomen. These muscles allow the diaphragm to function more efficiently, but are inactivated during rapid eye movement (REM) sleep thus decreasing respiratory efficiency (Muller & Bryan 1979).

The diaphragm and intercostal muscles of a neonate have a lower proportion of fatigue resistant fibres than the muscles of older infants and adults (Keens & Ianuzzo 1979). At 24 weeks' gestation they comprise only 10% of the total fibres, but these increase until the infant is 8 months old when the proportion of 50–60% is reached. This proportion is maintained throughout adult life. Premature or newborn infants are therefore particularly susceptible to fatigue if the work of breathing is increased. Apnoeic attacks or hypoventilation may result from diaphragmatic fatigue.

Most infants are obligatory nose-breathers for the first few months of life allowing the ability to feed and breathe simultaneously. This is probably related to the high position of the epiglottis and larynx which descend with age. This makes the neonate particularly vulnerable to nasal obstruction (Purcell 1976). The nasal airway offers high resistance to inspiration and therefore must be kept clear particularly in the presence of a nasogastric tube.

Any increase in the resistance to inspiration will considerably increase the work of breathing. Neonates cannot increase lung volume significantly compared to an adult and therefore must raise their respiratory rate in order to achieve an adequate minute ventilation. The normal respiratory rate in a neonate is in the range of 30–45 breaths per minute.

Neonates have a large number of small calibre airways which offer a high resistance to airflow. After the age of 5 years an increase in diameter of the small airways occurs, but until this time any disorder reducing the diameter of the small peripheral airways causes significant resistance to flow and small amounts of mucus can cause occlusion of the airways.

An increase in the work of breathing in an infant can be recognized by an increase in respiratory rate, nasal flaring (dilator nares is an accessory muscle of respiration) and subcostal, intercostal and sternal recession. The infant may grunt, closing the glottic muscles, in an attempt to increase his own positive expiratory pressure and thus prevent airway collapse (Pang & Mellins 1975).

The floppy chest wall does not counteract the elastic recoil of the lungs as does the more rigid adult structure. Therefore functional residual capacity (FRC) is low in infants. Any factors which decrease FRC will increase the work of breathing, for example atelectasis or the head-down position. This may affect the selection of treatment positions for physiotherapy. When atelectasis occurs it is hard for the infant to re-expand the collapsed alveoli because the compliant chest wall prevents the generation of adequate pleural pressures. Instead of increasing the respiratory work required to re-expand his lungs an infant may stop breathing (Gregory 1981). Attacks of apnoea are not uncommon.

The floppy chest wall is suggested as one of the reasons for ventilation being preferentially distributed to the uppermost lung in infants (p. 36). To obtain optimal oxygenation an infant with unilateral lung disease should be nursed with the unaffected lung uppermost (Davies *et al.* 1985). Conventional postural drainage positions may compromise the infant and care must be taken if using these positions. Normal arterial oxygen level at birth is 9·5 kPa (71 mmHg) and between 1 and 10 months it is in the range of 11–12 kPa (82–90 mmHg).

ASSESSMENT

Infants should never be treated 'routinely', but need careful and frequent assessment. The potential risks must be weighed against the possible benefits of treatment. It is often inappropriate to treat an acutely ill hypoxic infant as any handling at a critical stage may cause deterioration. If excess secretions are present and the decision has been made to treat an infant, close observation of clinical signs and monitoring equipment is essential to detect changes. Treatment may be altered or stopped according to these observations.

Before examining the patient, the physiotherapist will study the patient's history, chest radiographs and investigations recorded in the medical notes. Looking at the current progress charts the following questions will be considered:

1 Is he intubated and being ventilated on IPPV, IMV (intermittent mandatory ventilation), CPAP or is he self-ventilating? What is the respiratory rate?

2 What are the arterial blood gas results? Is the patient breathing air or oxygen?

3 What is the pulse and the arterial blood pressure? Hypotension and bradycardia can be signs of neonatal hypoxaemia. The normal blood pressure of an infant, less than 1 year, is between 60/35 and 70/40 and normal heart rate is 120 beats/minute. Tachycardia is considered to be a rate more than 180 and bradycardia less than 100 beats/minute.

4 What is the temperature? Toe temperature may be recorded as well as central temperature to give an indication of peripheral vasoconstriction and cardiac output.

5 What drugs is the patient being given and when was the last dose of any drug relevant to physiotherapy given?

On observation and examination of the patient the physiotherapist will consider further points:

1 Are any of the following signs present:
Nasal flaring
Grunting
Subcostal, intercostal or sternal recession
Hyperinflation of the chest
Cough
Stridor
Audible wheeze – inspiratory or expiratory?

2 Is movement of the chest symmetrical?

3 What is the patient's colour? Pale, grey, mottled? These are often signs of hypoxaemia and low cardiac output. Cyanosis is a sign of severe hypoxia, but it could be irrelevant if an infant has congenital heart disease.

4 On auscultation, are there crackles, wheezes, signs of consolidation or atelectasis? Listening to an infant's chest is difficult as sounds from the upper chest can be transmitted all over the chest. If the infant is crying it is still possible to listen during inspiration as the infant momentarily stops crying to breathe in.

5 Is the infant taking his feeds well or is he too breathless to feed adequately? Has he got an orogastric or nasogastric tube for feeding? It is important to find out the times that feeds will be given in order to plan to treat the infant before feeds.

PHYSIOTHERAPY TECHNIQUES

Appropriate techniques of physiotherapy vary according to the age of the infant or child as well as the individual condition.

Breathing techniques

It is not possible to introduce voluntary breathing techniques until the age of 2 or 3 years. As soon as the cooperation of the child can be gained the techniques described in Chapter 4 (p. 15) are used. Encouragement by using various games or pretending to smell the scent of a favourite flower may help and a simple incentive spirometer may promote inspiratory effort following surgery. Blowing bubbles or playing 'blow football' using a wide bore tube are popular games. Huffing (FET) can be taught using a peak expiratory flow mouthpiece (fig. 18, p. 23).

Positioning

Postural drainage for clearance of secretions is carried out in the appropriate specific positions using the techniques described (p. 23). In addition to the contra-indications listed (p. 30) abdominal distension may contra-indicate the head down drainage position as respiration will be compromised by decreasing functional residual capacity (FRC). The position should also be avoided in patients liable to elevation of intracranial pressure and following cardiac surgery until cardiac output is stabilized.

When not being positioned specifically for physiotherapy, infants with respiratory insufficiency should be positioned so that FRC and oxygen levels are enhanced. Lying with the head and shoulders raised allows the abdominal contents to fall and increases FRC. An infant often benefits from lying in the prone position with the head and shoulders elevated, the pressure exerted on the abdomen increases the efficiency of the diaphragm (Muller & Bryan 1979).

Hypoxic infants with unilateral lung disease should be nursed with the unaffected lung uppermost to gain optimal oxygenation (p. 36). Infants with unilateral air-trapping may benefit from the affected lung being dependent (Cohen *et al.* 1984).

Manual techniques

Mobilization of bronchial secretions may be assisted by clapping the chest wall. A skilled physiotherapist, using her finger tips or cupped hand (fig. 107), will be able to feel the chest more effectively than when using a percussive device. A small, cushioned face mask fitted on to the index or middle finger (fig. 108) has been shown to be a comfortable and effective method of chest percussion in infants (Tudehope & Bagley 1980). Physiotherapists can teach the nursing staff to give effective percussion using this device.

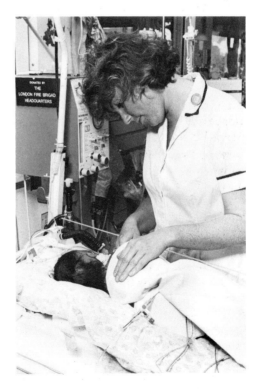

Fig. 107. *Chest clapping.*

149

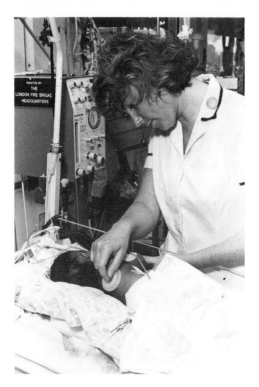

Fig. 108. *Chest percussion with cushioned face mask (Puritan–Bennett).*

An electric toothbrush has been used in an attempt to mobilize secretions, but no benefit has been shown (Tudehope & Bagley 1980) and infants sometimes appear upset by the application.

Manual vibrations with the fingers or hands may be useful when an infant's respiratory rate is slow enough to allow time to vibrate effectively throughout the expiratory phase. Care must be taken not to compress the chest wall too vigorously.

Techniques of percussion and vibration can be used with infants and children, both spontaneously breathing and when intubated and receiving assisted ventilation.

Inhalation of drugs

Devices and methods appropriate for inhalation of drugs are discussed with the treatment of asthma (p. 59) and cystic fibrosis (p. 67) and in the section on nebulization (p. 131).

Humidification

It is essential that ventilated infants are adequately humidified because the small endotracheal tube and/or small airways easily become blocked with tenacious secretions. This often leads to partial or total lung collapse. Gregory (1972) recommends that the inspired air should be 60–70% saturated at 37°C. The temperature probe should be positioned close to the patient on the inspiratory limb of the circuit to minimize the risk of thermal injury.

The extubated infant may also benefit from additional humidity particularly if oxygen therapy is required and secretions are tenacious. This may be administered via a headbox or mask. Care must be taken if using cold humidity, as this may cool the infant excessively. It may help if he wears a hat to minimize heat loss via the head.

Methods of humidification are discussed in Chapter 9 (p. 137).

Stimulus to coughing

Until a child is old enough to cough voluntarily, techniques have to be used to stimulate an effective cough when excess bronchial secretions are present.

Chest clapping often stimulates coughing and making a small child laugh, perhaps by tickling him, may also have the desired effect.

The trachea is soft and mobile in infants and young children. Intermittent lateral pressure on the trachea by the finger tips stimulates the cough reflex when the tracheal walls come into apposition. This is a simple and often effective technique which may avoid the necessity for naso-pharyngeal suction.

Suction of the non-intubated infant and child

Nasopharyngeal suction is often required during the treatment of infants and young children and must be carried out with great care to avoid unnecessary trauma to the mucus membranes. Oxygen should be turned on and available to apply, via a mask, immediately if the patient shows signs of hypoxia.

In addition to its use for stimulating the cough reflex, suction is used in infants to keep the nasal passages clear because they are usually obligatory nose breathers in the first few months of life (p. 147). If a nasogastric tube is in place, it is particularly important to select a small size of catheter so that the entire nasal airway is not blocked during the procedure.

The non-intubated patient should be positioned in side-lying to avoid the danger of inhalation of vomit. If an assistant is unavailable to hold him securely, he can be wrapped in a blanket with his arms inside as any wriggling movements make the procedure more difficult and more likely to cause trauma. The head and neck should be partially extended while inserting the catheter if difficulty is experienced reaching the pharynx. Sterile sachets of a water soluble jelly are sometimes used, but it is important not to block the nostril and dipping the catheter into sterile normal saline solution is preferable if any lubrication is required. Suction is carried out using a sterile technique.

To gauge the length of catheter to be inserted, in order to reach the pharynx, it is useful to measure the approximate distance from the anterior part of the ear to the patient's nose. In infants and young children the cough reflex can be stimulated in the pharynx. It is unnecessary and may be dangerous to insert the catheter into the trachea as laryngeal spasm may be induced.

Numerous types of catheter are available, but it is suggested that those with multiple side-holes cause less mucosal damage than those with a single side-hole (Young 1984). A system with a Y-connection or catheters with a control valve should be used to allow interrupted suction and to avoid a build-up of pressure during insertion of the catheter. Catheters without a Y-connection or control valve must be kinked during insertion, but the sudden release of the built-up pressure in an infant's airway is unacceptable.

The smallest diameter catheter that will effectively clear the secretions should be selected. If secretions are tenacious a catheter of slightly larger diameter will be required.

Vacuum pressure must not be unnecessarily high because tissue damage can be caused. In pre-term infants vacuum pressure should be limited to 80–100 mmHg and in older infants and children the pressure should be kept below 150 mmHg. It should be increased only if secretions are not being cleared, for example in the presence of a large plug of mucus.

Suction of the intubated infant and child

The type of catheter selected and vacuum pressure are similar for intubated and non-intubated patients. Suction should always be interrupted by use of a Y-connector or control valve and should only be carried out while withdrawing the catheter from the airway. The size of catheter should be no greater than half the internal diameter of the endotracheal tube. There is a danger of causing airway collapse and atelectasis if a larger sized catheter or high vacuum pressures are used (Young 1984).

Suction can cause bradycardia due to vagal stimulation or secondary to hypoxia. It is vital that the physiotherapist constantly watches the infant's colour and listens to the cardiac monitor for bradycardia. If the heart rate falls below 80/minute, suction should be stopped immediately and if on a continuous oxygen monitor, suction should be stopped if the arterial oxygen level falls to 6·6 kPa (50 mmHg) (Roberton 1986). In a fully ventilated premature infant the time for suction should not exceed 5 seconds and in the older infant 5–10 seconds. By rotating the catheter gently between the fingers, while withdrawing it from the endotracheal tube, suction can be carried out effectively in this short period of time. A hand ventilation set attached to oxygen should be ready during the suction procedure and if there is any sign of bradycardia, suction should be stopped immediately and oxygen should be delivered by hand ventilation. Manual inflation of the lungs with 100% oxygen, for up to 15 seconds following suction, may reverse any hypoxia or atelectasis caused by suction.

Normal saline solution may be inserted into the endotracheal tube before suction to assist mobilization of secretions. For an infant under 1 year, between 0.3 and 1 ml can be used, the quantity depending on the tenacity of the secretions.

Sterile technique is essential with a catheter being inserted into an endotracheal tube only once. Infants and young children are usually intubated with an uncuffed tube. Until puberty the cricoid ring forms a partial, natural cuff. An air leak is present, but trauma from pressure of the tube on the trachea is avoided. Nasopharyngeal and oral suction are required to clear the pharynx of secretions in addition to suction via the endotracheal tube.

Manual hyperinflation

Manual hyperinflation is a useful technique to assist mobilization and removal of excess bronchial secretions in intubated infants and children. It is contra-indicated if cardiac output is poor, in the presence of a pneumothorax, in infants with stiff lungs requiring high ventilation pressures and in pre-term infants because of the high risk of causing a pneumothorax.

If there are no contra-indications to treatment and atelectasis or excess bronchial secretions are present, the infant is positioned with the affected lobe uppermost. It is important to monitor closely the infant's colour and heart rate because this position may increase ventilation-perfusion imbalance.

It is likely that an intubated infant will have a nasotracheal tube in preference to an orotracheal tube (fig. 109). Firmer fixation of the nasotracheal tube is possible so that there is less risk of trauma to the mucus membrane than with an oral tube. Infants can extubate themselves more easily with an oral tube and trauma of repeated re-intubation may eventually lead to tracheal stricture. Other advantages of nasal intubation are that the infant is free to suck a dummy and can have good mouth care. The freedom of the mouth is important for normal development of feeding and speech.

Before manual hyperinflation, normal saline (0·5 ml for a small infant) can be instilled into the tube. If it is inserted into the top of an endotracheal tube, very little may reach the bronchi. When secretions are viscid it is more effective to fill a catheter with saline and leaving the syringe attached, insert it into the endotracheal tube as far as possible, withdraw it 1 cm (to ensure that it is above the carina) and then instil a further 0.5 ml of saline.

A rebreathing bag of suitable size (500 ml up to 1 year) is connected to a supply of oxygen (4–6 litres/minute for a 500 ml bag) and attached carefully to the endotracheal tube. The connection to the tube must be carefully supported to avoid trauma to the infant and kinking of the tube. Before using the hyperinflation technique a few rapid shallow breaths by manual inflation are given to allow the infant to settle and to take over his breathing if he is agitated. This will also create turbulence to distribute the instilled saline.

The physiotherapist should carefully watch the chest and abdominal movement before disconnecting the infant from the ventilator because the aim of the hyperinflation technique is to deliver a deeper breath, giving slightly greater movement of the chest and abdomen than when on the ventilator. By using a slow inflation, a high peak inspiratory pressure is avoided

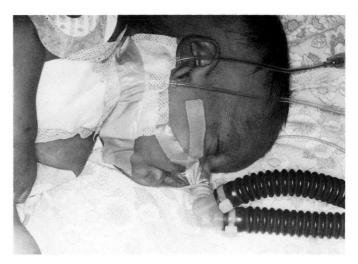

Fig. 109. *Intubated infant with nasotracheal tube.*

and the risk of causing a pneumothorax is lessened. A quick release of the bag gives a relatively high expiratory flow which assists mobilization of secretions. The rebreathing bag should not be emptied completely during the procedure, allowing a reservoir of gas and some positive end expiratory pressure to be maintained.

In infants with a high respiratory rate it may be necessary to give two or three quick tidal breaths with the bag followed by one hyperinflation instead of continuous hyperinflations. This will maintain adequate minute ventilation. If an infant is breathing spontaneously the manual hyperinflation should be synchronized with the inspiratory efforts.

When carrying out manual hyperinflation (fig. 110) the movement of the infant's chest and abdomen can be observed, but some physiotherapists find it useful to learn the techniques with a manometer fitted into the circuit. It is impossible to generalize about pressures needed for treatment, but as a guide the pressure given during manual hyperinfla-

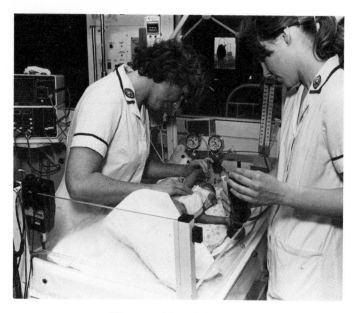

Fig. 110. *Manual hyperinflation with chest vibrations.*

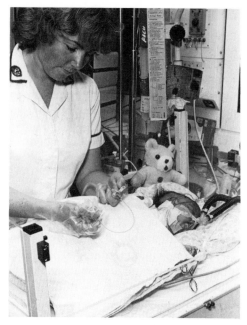

Fig. 111. *Preparing for suction.*

tion should be no more than an increase of 20% of the ventilator pressure. High inflation pressures may cause a pneumothorax and may compromise the cardiac output.

Chest percussion can be used in conjunction with manual hyperinflation or vibrations may be used during the expiratory phase. Suction is carried out after a short period of hyperinflation to clear the secretions that have been loosened (fig. 111). Throughout treatment it is vital to watch for any signs of a fall in cardiac output and to stop using hyperinflation if this occurs.

Following treatment, when the infant is re-connected to the ventilator, the physiotherapist should make certain that bilateral chest movement is present. It is possible that with movement of the infant the endotracheal tube may have slipped down into one of the main bronchi.

In most infants it is safe to use 100% oxygen to carry out manual hyperinflation, but it is contra-indicated in infants with duct dependent congenital heart defects as the oxygen may cause the duct to close. A mixture of air and oxygen should be used if manual hyperinflation is required.

If the child is agitated by manual hyperinflation, it is safer to treat him on the ventilator. Vibrations during the expiratory phase and percussion may be used, followed by suction as necessary.

THE PREMATURE OR LOW BIRTH WEIGHT INFANT

There are further problems in the pre-term infant which may influence the physiotherapist's treatment.

154

Temperature control

Pre-term infants have a large surface area for a small body mass. Heat loss (and gain) can be considerable. Maximal heat conservation is achieved in the foetal 'curled up' position, but sick neonates are frequently nursed supine in the 'frog' position with many surfaces exposed maximizing heat loss.

To maintain body temperature these infants have to utilize oxygen when they may already be in a hypoxic state. It is necessary to nurse them in a neutral, thermal environment where minimal oxygen consumption is required to maintain body temperature. This may be achieved by using incubators or over-head heaters and by maintaining the ambient room temperature at 27–28°C (Parker 1985). The physiotherapist must take care to maintain this temperature by preventing draughts, closing the incubator gently but as soon as possible and keeping the infant covered during treatment.

Infection

Premature infants are particularly susceptible to infection and the physiotherapist must be meticulous about hand washing. It is advisable to use the stethoscope provided for each patient as stethoscopes have been shown to be a source of cross infection (Gerken *et al.* 1972). Care must be taken when treating the infant to avoid damaging the very delicate skin.

Handling

It has already been stressed that suction can cause hypoxia, but in the sick premature infant any handling or disturbance will predispose to hypoxia and must be kept to a minimum.

Periventricular haemorrhage (PVH)

This used to be described as intraventricular haemorrhage (IVH). Sudden changes in arterial oxygen or carbon dioxide levels or blood pressure produce changes in cerebral blood flow. The friable capillaries in the rich vascular network on the floor of the lateral ventricles may rupture. Minimal handling will reduce the risk of hypoxic episodes and care must be taken to avoid blocking or dislodging the endotracheal tube. PVH is the major cause of death in very low birth weight infants especially in those who have been hypoxic, hypotensive or have had a pneumothorax or respiratory distress syndrome (Roberton 1986).

Physiotherapy

There must be a *definite indication* for treatment, for example excess bronchial secretions or atelectasis. Inappropriate or unnecessary physiotherapy may cause a marked deterioration in the infant's condition.

MEDICAL CONDITIONS

Respiratory distress syndrome (RDS)

Respiratory distress syndrome (hyaline membrane disease) is the most common neonatal respiratory disorder. It usually occurs in premature infants born before 37 weeks' gestation and is related to a deficiency of surfactant in the infant's lungs. Symptoms appear within 2 to 3 hours of birth and deterioration occurs over 24–36 hours as the infant tires.

Inadequate surfactant leads to progressive atelectasis. Lung compliance falls and the work of breathing increases. Hypoventilation causes a respiratory acidosis and together these factors result in severe hypoxaemia. Symptoms include a tachypnoea above 60 breaths/minute, grunting on expiration and subcostal, intercostal and sternal recession.

Research continues into the instillation or aerosol delivery of natural or synthetic surfactant into the lungs, but it is not yet a routinely available method of treatment. The aim of medical treatment is to provide adequate oxygenation to the infant until synthesis of his own surfactant becomes satisfactory, usually 36–48 hours after birth. Hypoxaemia inhibits the synthesis of surfactant and must be avoided.

Adequate oxygenation may be obtained by placing the infant in a headbox and supplying oxygen which is warmed and humidified. If more than 60% oxygen is needed to maintain the required oxygenation of between 8–12 kPa (60–90 mmHg), the infant will probably need ventilatory assistance by continuous positive airway pressure (CPAP) or intermittent positive pressure ventilation (IPPV).

Arterial oxygen levels are carefully maintained not only to avoid hypoxia, but also to minimize the risk of retinopathy of prematurity (retrolental fibroplasia). The capillaries of the premature retina may be affected by a level of oxygen above 16 kPa (120 mmHg). Proliferation of new capillaries, haemorrhage and fibrosis lead to severe visual impairment.

Excess bronchial secretions are rarely a problem with RDS and physiotherapy is unnecessary unless the infant develops a chest infection, or prolonged intubation results in production of secretions. If physiotherapy is required, manual hyperinflation is contra-indicated with premature lungs owing to the danger of creating a pneumothorax. Minimal handling is essential and the monitors must be carefully watched, during physiotherapy and suction, to avoid hypoxia and bradycardia.

Bronchopulmonary dysplasia

Bronchopulmonary dysplasia is a condition of the neonate which may result from prolonged artificial ventilation with a high concentration of inspired oxygen. Widespread destruction of alveoli leads to areas of collapse, emphysema and eventually to fibrosis. Oxygen therapy, IPPV with minimal peak inspiratory pressure or negative pressure ventilation may be required for many months until new alveoli develop. Viral and bacterial chest infections are common during this period and physiotherapy is required to avoid further lung damage.

Pneumonia

Congenital Pneumonia may occur as a result of inhalation of infected amniotic fluid. It is suspected in an infant where the mother is pyrexial and has had ruptured membranes for more than 12 hours. The infant shows signs of respiratory distress in the first few hours of life. The chest radiograph shows patchy shadowing often indistinguishable from RDS.

Aspiration pneumonia may be caused by aspiration of meconium just before birth or by aspiration of feeds in premature infants in whom sucking, swallowing and cough reflexes are poorly developed. Treatment for both these conditions is with oxygen and antibiotics. If excess bronchial secretions are present, appropriate postural drainage is carried out with careful monitoring (p. 149).

Viral and bacterial pneumonia. Viral pneumonia is more common than bacterial pneumonia in infants and children. Symptoms start with coryza (runny nose) and this is followed by cough, tachypnoea and difficulty with feeding. Bilateral bronchopneumonia is more common than lobar pneumonia. Postural drainage is indicated if excess bronchial secretions are present.

Acute bronchiolitis

Acute bronchiolitis is a common respiratory illness of infancy caused by a viral infection, predominantly the respiratory syncytial virus. It is most common in infants less than 1 year old with the peak occurrence between 2 and 4 months of age. Symptoms start with coryza and are followed by acute wheeze, rib and subcostal recession with tachypnoea, hyperinflation of the chest, cough and possible cyanosis. On auscultation fine crackles are heard throughout the lung fields. The condition usually progresses over 2 to 3 days and then improvement begins.

The infant is nursed with humidified oxygen, usually in a head box and is positioned with the head and shoulders raised or in the sitting position, to assist ventilation (p. 149). Nasal suction is necessary to keep the nasal passages as clear as possible. Intravenous feeding may be required as the infant may be too short of breath to feed adequately.

Physiotherapy is contra-indicated in the first 24–48 hours during the stage of acute respiratory distress. Handling should be minimal in the acute stage to try to avoid increasing hypoxia. Postural drainage is carried out during the recovery phase if excess bronchial secretions or areas of atelectasis are present. Following a study in patients with acute bronchiolitis Webb *et al.* (1985) recommended that physiotherapy should not be used routinely.

Pertussis (whooping cough)

Whooping cough is a common viral infectious disease of childhood. Coryza is followed by a paroxysmal cough which may persist for several weeks. The inspiratory 'whoop' often causes the child to vomit. Hypoxia is produced by the paroxysmal coughing and by aspiration of vomit. Attacks of apnoea may occur.

Postural drainage is contra-indicated in the acute stage because stimulation of coughing may induce further hypoxia. In the later stages postural drainage is required if there is persistent lobar collapse. Collapse of the right middle lobe is most common, probably because collateral ventilation to this lobe is ineffective in children (Inners *et al.* 1978). Parents should be instructed in postural drainage techniques which should be carried out before meals.

Laryngo-tracheobronchitis (croup) and epiglottitis

Laryngo-tracheobronchitis is usually caused by a virus and is common in children between the ages of 1 and 5 years. Coryza is followed by a 'barking' cough and stridor. Steroids may be prescribed to reduce the oedema in the airway. The child is nursed with high humidification and may require intubation if adequate ventilation cannot be maintained. If a very small endotracheal tube is used, mechanical ventilation may be necessary.

Epiglottitis is a dangerous condition of sudden onset usually occurring between the ages of 3 and 7 years. Sore throat, dyspnoea and difficulty in swallowing develop, but in contrast to laryngo-tra-cheobronchitis there is no 'barking' cough. The sudden inflammatory changes can cause closure of the epiglottis, requiring an emergency tracheotomy. IPPV may be necessary if the tracheal tube is very small.

Physiotherapy is not indicated in the treatment of these conditions unless the child is intubated and secretions cannot be cleared adequately with endotracheal suction.

Inhalation of a foreign body

Inhalation of foreign bodies, for example small toys or peanuts, is common throughout infancy and childhood. Most foreign bodies lodge in the main bronchi, the right side slightly more often than the left. If the foreign body is not immediately coughed out, it will cause obstruction or partial obstruction of the airway and may lead to underlying atelectasis. Bronchoscopy is carried out as soon as possible to remove the offending object and postural drainage should be started soon after the bronchoscopy to gain re-expansion of any atelectatic areas.

Oil in peanuts causes an inflammatory reaction in the airways, the child may be febrile and recovery may be slower than with other foreign bodies.

Neuromuscular disorders

Weakness of the respiratory muscles may occur in neuromuscular disorders such as Duchenne muscular dystrophy and spinal muscular atrophy. With a decrease in vital capacity and weakness of the muscles of

expiration, clearance of tracheobronchial secretions is ineffective. Atelectasis and respiratory tract infections may result. Prophylactic breathing exercises and postural drainage should be carried out regularly. IPPB or PCPAP may be useful adjuncts (p. 120 & p. 129).

Asthma (p. 55) and cystic fibrosis (p. 64)

These respiratory conditions require physiotherapy and are discussed with the treatment of adults.

SURGICAL CONDITIONS

Congenital cardiac defects

Palliative operations may be carried out in children too young for corrective surgery or where the heart is anatomically unsuitable. These operations include banding of the pulmonary artery and the Blalock--Taussig shunt.

The corrective operations commonly performed in infants and children with congenital cardiac defects include: ligation of patent ductus arteriosus, resection of coarctation of the aorta, open pulmonary or aortic valvotomy, closure of atrial and ventricular septal defects, total correction of Fallot's tetralogy, arterial switch or Mustard's operation for transposition of the great arteries, correction of anomalous pulmonary venous drainage, Fontan procedure for tricuspid atresia (absent right atrio-ventricular connection), the Rastelli procedure for pulmonary atresia and correction of truncus arteriosus.

For any infant or child undergoing

cardiac surgery, the principles of physiotherapy are similar. Assessment of the respiratory state is important before surgery if possible and at frequent intervals in the post-operative stage.

PRE-OPERATIVE TRAINING

The amount of pre-operative training in children depends on their age. As well as teaching the child, it is important to explain the necessity of the exercises to the parents who are often with their children for long periods of the day and can encourage practice.

Infants with cardiac defects (with left to right shunt) often have increased pulmonary blood flow and excessive bronchial secretions. These infants are susceptible to repeated chest infections. Physiotherapy may be necessary pre-operatively to clear excess secretions. Treatment consists of modified postural drainage, percussion and/or gentle vibrations and nasopharyngeal suction to stimulate coughing.

Children 18 months–3 years can be taught breathing exercises by means of blowing bubbles or paper tissues. If excess bronchial secretions are present pre-operatively, postural drainage can probably be performed (with the doctor's permission) and clapping of the chest usually stimulates coughing.

Children over 3 years are taught lower thoracic expansion exercises, the forced expiration technique and coughing. An incentive spirometer may be useful to emphasize inspiration. Postural drainage is performed if necessary. Arm movements are encouraged by clapping the hands over the head and for children over 5 years old, more shoulder girdle and arm exercises are included.

POST-OPERATIVE TREATMENT

Many infants and children are intubated and mechanically ventilated post-operatively (fig. 112). Careful assessment of the patient (p. 147) before each treatment is essential. If the cardiovascular state is stable and excess bronchial secretions or areas of atelectasis are present, manual hyperinflation may be indicated (p. 152). Saline is instilled into the endotracheal tube before manual hyperinflation. Clapping or vibrations may be carried out with the hyperinflations and endotracheal, nasal and oral suction are used to clear secretions (p. 152). Positioning of the patient will depend on the cardiovascular state.

If manual hyperinflation is contra-indicated, but excess bronchial secretions are present, clapping and/or vibrations in time with the ventilator may be carried out, followed by suction.

The heart is often oedematous immediately following surgery and insertion of

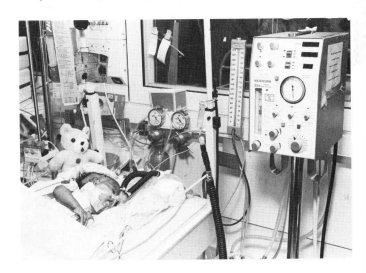

Fig. 112. *Mechanical ventilation.*

159

conduit is necessary in some procedures. The heart requires extra space in both these circumstances and the surgeon may leave the chest 'open' with the sternum splinted for a few days. If the heart is constricted by the chest wall, cardiac output may be impaired. During this period manual hyperinflation may be indicated if excess secretions are present, but clapping and vibrations are omitted.

Intermittent mandatory ventilation (IMV) and continuous positive airway pressure (CPAP) are frequently used in the transition between IPPV and extubation. It has been shown that, following cardiac surgery in infants, the functional residual capacity (FRC) is reduced and that CPAP causes the FRC to rise towards the normal (Gregory *et al.* 1975). When compliance is reduced following open heart surgery, CPAP results in a significant increase in Pao_2.

Physiotherapy with manual hyperinflation can be used when the patient is nursed on IMV or CPAP. It is particularly important to synchronize the hyperinflations with the patient's inspiratory efforts and if he becomes agitated it is advisable to omit this and use clapping, vibrations and suction while connected to the IMV or CPAP circuit.

When the child is first transferred from IPPV to spontaneous ventilation with CPAP, disturbance by physiotherapy during the first 2 hours should be avoided unless bronchial secretions are excessive.

Following the removal of pleural drains, a radiograph is taken to exclude a pneumothorax. Manual hyperinflations should be postponed until after this radiograph, but if excessive secretions are present treatment can be carried out with the patient on the ventilator in the intervening period.

Radiographic appearances of the chest may be misleading to the physiotherapist. With a left to right cardiac shunt there is an increase in pulmonary vascular markings bilaterally. Following a Blalock-Taussig shunt there is a unilateral increase in pulmonary vascular markings. The increased shadowing in these instances may be confused with respiratory infection. The lower lobe of the left lung may be collapsed as a result of mechanical compression by the enlarged heart and enlarged blood vessels.

Suction catheters are likely to enter the right upper lobe bronchus because of the anatomy of the bronchial tree. Poor suction technique may withdraw air from the upper lobe and trauma to the airways can cause oedema. Both these factors predispose to atelectasis.

After the patient has been extubated or with non-intubated infants and children, modified postural drainage is carried out using breathing techniques if the child is old enough to cooperate, clapping and gentle vibrations. Appropriate methods of stimulating a cough are used (p. 150).

Infants are often nursed in a head box with high humidification and oxygen (fig. 113). During treatment, when the head box is removed, oxygen should be turned on and available to apply via a mask if signs of hypoxia are observed.

When atelectasis of part or the whole of a lung has occurred and is not responding to physiotherapy the patient can be temporarily intubated to allow effective inflation and suction during physiotherapy. Older children may respond well to IPPB or PCPAP (p. 129), with a mask or mouthpiece, in conjunction with physiotherapy.

As soon as the child is allowed out of bed, mobility helps to stimulate deep breathing and coughing. Many children have no problems with excess secretions after cardiac surgery, but some develop poor posture and are reluctant to move. Exercises to encourage mobility and posture correction are given.

The frequency of treatment in the infant or child post-operatively depends on the individual patient's condition. Assessment is essential to determine whether treatment is indicated or contra-indicated and to evaluate the effects of treatment. If secretions or atelectasis are present and the cardiovascular state is stable, 2-hourly treatment is often necessary.

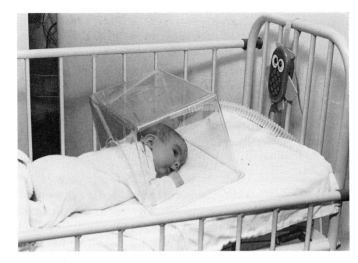

Fig. 113. *An infant in a headbox.*

Pulmonary surgery

Pulmonary surgery is rarely performed in infants, but when it is necessary the principles of physiotherapy are the same as for cardiac surgery. For older children undergoing pulmonary surgery, treatment is similar to that for adults (p. 79).

Congenital diaphragmatic hernia

In this disorder the diaphragm does not fuse completely and bowel herniates into the chest preventing the lungs from fully expanding. The infant will probably show signs of respiratory distress and may require endotracheal intubation and mechanical ventilation. Surgery is carried out as soon as possible to reposition the bowel in the abdomen and repair the diaphragmatic defect. There is usually pulmonary hypoplasia in association with congenital diaphragmatic hernia and IPPV may be required for several weeks.

Physiotherapy is indicated only if there are excess bronchial secretions. The pulmonary hypoplasia may predispose to

pneumothorax and manual hyperinflation may be contra-indicated.

Oesophageal atresia and tracheo-oesophageal fistula

The most common congenital defect of the oesophagus is with the upper portion of the oesophagus ending in a blind pouch and a fistula between the upper trachea and lower oesophagus (fig. 114).

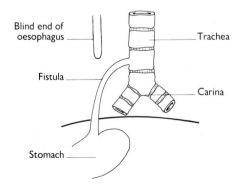

Blind end of oesophagus

Trachea

Fistula

Carina

Stomach

Fig. 114. *Diagram of the most common form of oesophageal atresia with trache-oesophageal fistula.*

161

The infant is unable to swallow oral secretions and noisy breathing with mucus regurgitating from the mouth is observed soon after birth. The first feed will cause acute choking, coughing and cyanosis (Kelnar & Harvey 1981).

Until corrective surgery can be undertaken the upper portion of the oesophagus must be suctioned continuously to prevent aspiration into the lungs and the infant may be fed intravenously or by gastrostomy. He is nursed in the prone position or on his side and when suction of saliva is adequately established the head-up position will prevent reflux of gastric contents via the trache-oesophageal fistula.

The tracheal fistula is closed through a right thoracotomy and a primary anastamosis of the two parts of the oesophagus is made where possible. In a minority of cases the anatomy of the oesophagus makes this impossible and the fistula is repaired and cervical oesophagostomy and a feeding gastrotomy are established. Reconstruction of the oesophagus is undertaken at a later date by colonic interposition.

Physiotherapy may be required pre-operatively to assist clearance of excess bronchial secretions and aspirated material, if pulmonary complications have already occurred. Post-operatively the infant may be mechanically ventilated and if necessary physiotherapy should be given to clear secretions when intubated and after extubation. Nasopharyngeal suction must be carried out with care, avoiding the catheter entering the oesophagus and trauma at the site of the oesophageal anastamosis.

The infant is nursed with his head elevated for the first few days to avoid stress at the suture line and assist healing. The head-down position should not be used at any stage because reflux of gastic contents may occur. It has been shown that many of these patients have low oesophageal sphincter pressures and are likely to have reflux. An anti-reflux surgical procedure may be carried out (Ashmore 1982).

References

Andersen D.H. (1938) Cystic fibrosis of the pancreas and its relation to celiac disease. A clinical and pathological study. *American Journal of Diseases of the Child.* **56**, 344–99.

Andersen J.B. & Klausen N.O. (1982) A new mode of administration of nebulized bronchodilator in severe bronchospasm. *European Journal of Respiratory Diseases*, suppl. **119**(63), 97–100.

Andersen J.B., Olesen K.P., Eikard B. *et al.* (1980) Periodic continuous positive airway pressure, CPAP, by mask in the treatment of atelectasis. *European Journal of Respiratory Diseases.* **61**, 20–5.

Asbury A.J. (1985) Patients' memories and reactions to intensive care. *Care of the critically ill* **1**(2), 12–13.

Ashmore P.G. (1982) In *Oesophageal and Other Thoracic Problems*, p. 132 (ed. W.G. Williams & R.E. Smith). Wright PSG, Bristol.

Ayres S.M., Kozam R.L. & Lukas, D.S. (1963) The effects of intermittent positive pressure breathing on intrathoracic pressure, pulmonary mechanics and the work of breathing. *American Review of Respiratory Disease.* **87**, 370–9.

Banner, N.R. & Govan, J.R. (1986) Long term transtracheal oxygen delivery through microcatheter in patients with hypoxaemia due to chronic obstructive airways disease. *British Medical Journal.* **293**, 111–14.

Bateman J.R.M., Newman S.P., Daunt K.M. *et al.* (1979) Regional lung clearance of excessive bronchial secretions during chest physiotherapy in patients with stable chronic airways obstruction. *Lancet*, **i**, 294–7.

Batten J.C. & Matthew D. J. (1983) The respiratory system, in *Cystic Fibrosis* 125–7 (eds M.E. Hodson, A.P. Norman & J.C. Batten). Baillière Tindall, London.

Bethune D.D. (1975) Neurophysiological facilitation of respiration in the unconscious adult patient. *Physiotherapy Canada.* **27** (**5**), 241–5.

Bigby T.D., Margolskee D., Curtis J.L. *et al.* (1986) The usefulness of induced sputum in the diagnosis of Pneumocystis carinii pneumonia in patients with acquired immunodeficiency syndrome. *American Review of Respiratory Disease.* **133**, 515–18.

Booker H., Harries D., Rehahn M. & Collins J. (1985) Progressive exercise training: subjective and objective changes. *Physiotherapy Practice.* **1**, 31–6.

Brambilla C., Levy P., Lepaulle B. *et al.* (1987) Ambulatory monitoring in COPD patients using portable oxymeters. *Thorax.* **42**(3), 216 (abstract).

Branthwaite M.A. (1980) *Artificial Ventilation for Pulmonary Disease*, 2nd ed. Pitman Medical, Tonbridge.

Butland R.J.A., Pang J., Gross E.R. *et al.* (1982) Two-, six-, and 12-minute walking tests in respiratory disease. *British Medical Journal.* **284**, 1607–8.

Campbell A.H., O'Connell J.M. & Wilson F. (1975) The effect of chest physiotherapy upon the FEV_1 in chronic bronchitis. *Medical Journal of Australia.* **1**, 33–5.

Carroll N. & Branthwaite M.A. (1988) Control of nocturnal hypoventilation by nasal intermittent positive pressure ventilation. *Thorax.* In press.

Chang N., Levison H., Cunningham K. *et al.* (1973) An evaluation of nightly mist tent therapy for patients with cystic fibrosis. *American Review of Respiratory Disease.* **107**, 672–5.

Clay M.M. & Clarke S.W. (1987) Effect of nebulized aerosol size on lung deposition in patients with mild asthma. *Thorax.* **42**(3), 190–4.

Clay M. M., Pavia D., Newman S.P. *et al.* (1983) Assessment of jet nebulizers for lung aerosol therapy. *Lancet.* **ii**, 592–4.

Cleeton C.A. (1978) A nurse's guide to intra-aortic balloon assistance. *Nursing Times.* **74**, 1890–5.

Clement A.J. & Hübsch S.K. (1968) Chest physiotherapy by the 'bag squeezing' method. *Physiotherapy.* **54**(10), 355–9.

Cochrane G.M., Webber B.A. & Clarke S.W. (1977) Effects of sputum on pulmonary function. *British Medical Journal.* **2**, 1181–3.

Cohen R.S., Smith D.W., Stevenson D.K. *et al.* (1984) Lateral decubitus position as therapy for persistent focal pulmonary interstitial emphysema in neonates: a preliminary report. *Journal of Pediatrics.* **104**, 441–3.

Comroe J.H. (1965) *Physiology of Respiration.* Year Book Medical Publishers Incorporated, p. 122.

Connors A.F., Hammon W.E., Martin R.J. & Rogers R.M. (1980) Chest physical therapy: the immediate effect on oxygenation in acutely ill patients. *Chest.* **78**(4), 559–64.

Cooke J.C., Currie D.C., Morgan A.D. *et al.* (1987) Role of computed tomography in diagnosis of bronchiectasis. *Thorax.* **42**, 272–7.

Craig D.B. (1981) Postoperative recovery of pulmonary function. *Anesthesia and Analgesia.***60**(1), 46–52.

Dail C.W. (1951) Glossopharyngeal breathing by paralyzed patients. *California Medicine.* **75**(3), 217–8.

Dail C.W., Affeldt J.E. & Collier C.R. (1955) Clinical aspects of glossopharyngeal breathing. *Journal of the American Medical Association.* **158**, 445–9.

Davies H., Kitchman R., Gordon I. & Helms P. (1985) Regional ventilation in infancy. *New England Journal of Medicine.* **313**, 1626–8.

Dean E. (1985) Effect of body position on pulmonary function. *Physical therapy.* **65**(5), 613–8.

De Troyer A. & Estenne M. (1984) Coordination between rib cage muscles and diaphragm during quiet breathing in humans. *Journal of Applied Physiology.* **57**(3), 899–906.

De Troyer A., Kelly S. & Zin W.A. (1983) Mechanical action of the intercostal muscles on the ribs. *Science.* **220**, 87–8.

Donaldson A. & Gandevia B. (1962) The physiotherapy of emphysema. *Australian Journal of Physiotherapy.* **8**(2), 55–69.

du Bois R.M., McAllister W.A.C. & Branthwaite M.A. (1983) Alveolar proteinosis: diagnosis and treatment over a 10-year period. *Thorax.* **38**, 360–3.

Ellis E.R., Bye P.T.P., Bruderer J.W. & Sullivan C.E. (1987) Treatment of respiratory failure during sleep in patients with neuromuscular disease. *American Review of Respiratory Disease.* **135**, 148–52.

Escobedo M.B. (1982) Fetal and neonatal cardiopulmonary physiology, in *Practical Neonatal Respiratory Care* (ed. R.L. Schreiner & J.A. Kisling), 1–18. Raven Press, New York.

Evans T.W., Waterhouse J. & Howard P. (1983) Clinical experience with the oxygen concentrator. *British Medical Journal.* **287**, 459–61.

Falk M., Kelstrup M., Andersen J.B. *et al.* (1984) Improving the ketchup bottle method with positive expiratory pressure, PEP, in cystic fibrosis. *European Journal of Respiratory Diseases.* **65**, 423–32.

Fitch K.D. & Morton A.R. (1971) Specificity of exercise in exercise-induced asthma. *British Medical Journal.* **4**, 577–81.

Fixley M.S., Roussos C.S., Murphy B. *et al.* (1978) Flow dependence of gas distribution and the pattern of inspiratory muscle contraction. *Journal of Applied Physiology.* **45**, 733–41.

Flenley D.C. (1985) Short review: inspiratory muscle training. *European Journal of Respiratory Diseases.* **67**, 153–8.

Fletcher C., Peto R., Tinker C. & Speizer F.E. (1976) *The Natural History of Chronic Bronchitis and Emphysema.* 146–7. Oxford University Press, Oxford.

Forgacs P. (1978) *Lung Sounds.* Baillière Tindall, London.

Gandevia B. (1963) The spirogram of gross expiratory tracheobronchial collapse in emphysema. *Quarterly Journal of Medicine, New Series XXXII.* **125**, 23–31.

George R.J.D., Johnson M.A., Pavia D. *et al.* (1985a) Increase in mucociliary clearance in normal man induced by oral high frequency oscillation. *Thorax.* **40**, 433–7.

George R.J.D., Winter R.J.D., Johnson M.A. *et al.* (1985b) Effect of oral high frequency ventilation by jet or oscillator on minute ventilation in normal subjects. *Thorax.* **40**, 749–55.

Gerken A., Cavanagh S. & Winner H.I. (1972) Infection hazard from stethoscopes in hospital. *Lancet,* **i**, 1214–5.

Gherini S., Peters R. M. & Virgilio R.W. (1979) Mechanical work on the lungs and work of breathing with positive end-expiratory pressure and continuous positive airway pressure. *Chest.* **76**, 251–6.

Gibson G.J., Edmonds J.P. & Hughes G.R.V. (1977) Diaphragm function and lung involvement in systemic lupus erythematosus. *American Journal of Medicine.* **63**, 926–32.

Gormezano J. and Branthwaite M.A. (1972a) Effects

of physiotherapy during intermittent positive pressure ventilation. *Anaesthesia.* **27**, 258–64.

Gormezano J. & Branthwaite M.A. (1972b) Pulmonary physiotherapy with assisted ventilation. *Anaesthesia.* **27**, 249–57.

Grant R. (1970) The physiological basis for increased exercise ability in patients with emphysema, after breathing and exercise training (a review of the literature) *Physiotherapy.* **56**(12), 541–7.

Green M. & Moxham J. (1985) The respiratory muscles. *Clinical Science.* **68**, 1–10.

Gregory G.A. (1972) Respiratory care of newborn infants. *Pediatric Clinics of North America.* **19**, 311–24.

Gregory G.A. (ed.) (1981) *Respiratory Failure in the Child.* p. vii Churchill Livingstone, New York.

Gregory G.A., Edmunds L.H., Kitterman J.A. *et al.* (1975) Continuous positive airway pressure and pulmonary and circulatory function after cardiac surgery in infants less than three months of age. *Anesthesiology.* **43**, 426–31.

Grimby G., Oxhøj H. & Bake B. (1975) Effects of abdominal breathing in distribution of ventilation in obstructive lung disease. *Clinical Science and Molecular Medicine.* **48**, 193–9.

Gross D., Ladd H.W., Riley E.J. *et al.* (1980) The effect of training on strength and endurance of the diaphragm in quadriplegia. *American Journal of Medicine.* **68**, 27–35.

Gunawardena K.A., Patel B., Campbell I.A. *et al.* (1984) Oxygen as a driving gas for nebulisers: safe or dangerous? *British Medical Journal.* **288**, 272–4.

Hakim M. & Wallwork J. (1985) Heart-lung transplantation. *Hospital update.* **11**(9), 653–63.

Hartley J.P.R. (1979) Exercise-induced asthma (editorial) *Thorax.* **34**, 571–4.

Higgens J.M. (1966) The management in cabinet respirators of patients with acute or residual respiratory muscle paralysis. *Physiotherapy.* **52**, 425–30.

Hodson M.E., Penketh A.R.L. & Batten J.C. (1981) Aerosol carbenicillin and gentamicin treatment of pseudomonas aeruginosa infection in patients with cystic fibrosis. *Lancet.* **ii**, 1137–9.

Hofmeyr J.L., Webber B.A. & Hodson M.E. (1986) Evaluation of positive expiratory pressure as an adjunct to chest physiotherapy in the treatment of cystic fibrosis. *Thorax.* **41**, 951–4.

Hooper A.E.T. (1967) Physical therapy for an emphysematous patient. *Proceedings of the 5th WCPT International Congress,* 119–33.

Hough A. (1986) How does head injury influence the physiotherapy management of the ventilated patient? *ACPRC Newsletter.* **9**, 25–33.

Howard P., Cayton R. M., Brennan S.R. & Anderson P.B. (1977) Lignocaine aerosol and persistent cough. *British Journal of Diseases of the Chest.* **71**, 19–24.

Inners C.R., Terry P.B., Traystman R.J. & Menkes H.A. (1978) Collateral ventilation and the middle lobe syndrome. *American Review of Respiratory Disease.* **118**, 305–10.

Innocenti D. (1987) Chronic hyperventilation syndrome, 536–49. In *Cash's Textbook for Chest, Heart and Vascular Disorders for Physiotherapists* 4th ed (ed. P.A. Downie) Faber & Faber, London.

Innocenti D. (1986) Handling the critically ill patient. *Physiotherapy.* **72**(3) 125–8.

Intermittent Positive Pressure Breathing Trial Group (1983) Intermittent positive pressure breathing therapy of chronic obstructive pulmonary disease. *Annals of Internal Medicine.* **99**, 612–20.

Keens T.G. & Ianuzzo C.D. (1979) Development of fatigue-resistant muscle fibers in human ventilatory muscles. *American Review of Respiratory Disease,* suppl. **119**, 139–41.

Kelleher W.H. & Parida R.K. (1957) Glossopharyngeal breathing. *British Medical Journal.* **2**, 740–3.

Kelnar C.J. & Harvey D. (1981) *The Sick Newborn Baby.* Baillière Tindall, London.

Kilham H., Tooley M. & Silverman M. (1979) Running, walking, and hyperventilation causing asthma in children. *Thorax.* **34**, 582–6.

Lafortuna C.L. & Fazio F. (1984) Acute effect of inhaled salbutamol on mucociliary clearance in health and chronic bronchitis. *Respiration.* **45**, 111–23.

Langlands J. (1967) The dynamics of cough in health and in chronic bronchitis. *Thorax.* **22**, 88–96.

Last R.J. (1972) *Anatomy, Regional and Applied* 5th ed. Churchill, London.

Lehrer S. (1984) *Understanding Lung Sounds.* W.B. Saunders, Philadelphia.

Leith D. (1968) Cough. *Physical Therapy.* **48**, 439–47.

Lightbody I.M., Ingram C.G., Legge J.S. & Johnston R.N. (1978) Ipratropium bromide, salbutamol and prednisolone in bronchial asthma and chronic bronchitis. *British Journal of Diseases of the Chest.* **72**, 181–6.

Loddenkemper R. (1975) Dose- and time-response of Sch 1000 MDI on total (R_t) and expiratory

(R_e) airways resistance in patients with chronic bronchitis and emphysema. *Postgraduate Medical Journal.* **51**, suppl. 7, 97.

Mallinson B.M., Burgess D.A., Cockroft C. & David T. J. (1981) Exercise training for children with asthma. *Physiotherapy.* **67**, 106–8.

Martin C.J., Ripley H., Reynolds J. & Best F. (1976) Chest physiotherapy and the distribution of ventilation. *Chest.* **69**, 174–8.

Matthews H.R. & Hopkinson R.B. (1984) Treatment of sputum retention by minitracheotomy. *British Journal of Surgery.* **71**, 147–50.

Matthews L.W., Doershuk C.F., Wise M. *et al.* (1964) A therapeutic regimen for patients with cystic fibrosis. *Journal of Pediatrics.* **65**, 558–75.

May D.B. & Munt P.W. (1979) Physiologic effects of chest percussion and postural drainage in patients with stable chronic bronchitis. *Chest.* **75**(1), 29–32.

McCool F.D., Mayewski R.F., Shayne D.S. *et al.* (1986) Intermittent positive pressure breathing in patients with respiratory muscle weakness *Chest.* **90**(4) 546–52.

McGavin C.R. (1976) A modified aerosol inhaler for teaching technique. *Lancet.* **ii**, 1227.

McGavin C.R., Gupta S.P., Lloyd E.L. & McHardy G.J.R. (1977) Physical rehabilitation for the chronic bronchitic: results of a controlled trial of exercises in the home. *Thorax.* **32**, 307–11.

McGavin C.R., Gupta S.P. & McHardy G.J.R. (1976a) Twelve-minute walking test for assessing disability in chronic bronchitis. *British Medical Journal.* **1**, 822–3.

McGavin C.R., Naoe H. & McHardy G.J.R. (1976b) Does inhalation of salbutamol enable patients with airway obstruction to walk further? *Clinical Science and Molecular Medicine.* **51**, 12–13.

Mead J., Takishima T. & Leith D. (1970) Stress distribution in lungs: a model of pulmonary elasticity. *Journal of Applied Physiology.* **28**, 596–608.

Mead J., Turner J.M., Macklem P.T. & Little J.B. (1967) Significance of the relationship between lung recoil and maximum expiratory flow. *Journal of Applied Physiology.* **22**, 95–108.

Medical Research Council (1965) Definition and classification of chronic bronchitis for clinical and epidemiological purposes. *Lancet.* **i**, 775–9.

Medical Research Council Working Party (1981) Long term domiciliary oxygen therapy in chronic hypoxic cor pulmonale complicating chronic bronchitis and emphysema. *Lancet.* **i**, 681–6.

Menkes H.A. & Britt J. (1980) Rationale for physical therapy. *American Review of Respiratory Disease.* **122**, suppl. part 2, 127–31.

Menkes H.A. & Traystman R.J. (1977) Collateral ventilation. *American Review of Respiratory Disease.* **116**, 287–309.

Miller D.L. (1963) A study of techniques for the examination of sputum in a field survey of chronic bronchitis. *American Review of Respiratory Disease.* **88**, 473–83.

Mitchell D.M., Solomon M.A., Tolfree S.E.J. *et al.* (1987) Effect of particle size of bronchodilator aerosols on lung distribution and pulmonary function in patients with chronic asthma. *Thorax.* **42**, 457–61.

Moon M.H. (1981) Biofeedback using a respiration parameter in the treatment of behavioural breathing disorders. *New Zealand Journal of Physiotherapy.* **9**(2) 19–20.

Morgan M.D.L., Silver J.R. & Williams S.J. (1986) The respiratory system of the spinal cord patient in *Management of Spinal Cord Injuries* (eds R.F. Bloch & M. Basbaum). Williams & Wilkins, USA.

Morran C.G., Finlay I.G., Mathieson M. *et al.* (1983) Randomized controlled trial of physiotherapy for postoperative pulmonary complications. *British Journal of Anaesthesia.* **55**, 1113–7.

Mosley S. (1985) *The Use of Tank Ventilators at the Brompton Hospital.* Brompton Hospital, London.

Muller N.L. & Bryan A.C. (1979) Chest wall mechanics and respiratory muscles in infants. *Pediatric Clinics of North America.* **26**(3), 503–16.

Mungall I.P.F. & Hainsworth R. (1979) Assessment of respiratory function in patients with chronic obstructive airways disease. *Thorax.* **34**, 254–8.

Myles P.V. (1970) Use of the entonox machine in post-operative chest physiotherapy. *Physiotherapy.* **56**, 559–60.

Newman S.P. & Clarke S.W. (1983) Therapeutic aerosols 1—physical and practical considerations. *Thorax.* **38**, 881–6.

Newman S.P., Pellow P.G.D. & Clarke S.W. (1986) Droplet size distributions of nebulised aerosols for inhalation therapy. *Clinical Physics and Physiological Measurement.* **7**, 139–46.

Nocturnal Oxygen Therapy Trial Group (1980) Continuous or nocturnal oxygen therapy in hypoxemic chronic obstructive lung disease: a clinical trial. *Annals of Internal Medicine.* **93**, 391–8.

O'Neill P.A., Dodd M., Phillips B. *et al.* (1987) Regular exercise and reduction of breathlessness in patients with cystic fibrosis. *British Journal of Diseases of the Chest.* **81**, 62–9.

Orenstein D.M., Henke K.G. and Cerny F.J. (1983) Exercise and cystic fibrosis. *The Physician and Sports Medicine.* **11**(1), 57–63.

Pang L.M. & Mellins R.B. (1975) Neonatal cardio-respiratory physiology. *Anesthesiology.* **43**(2), 171–96.

Parker A.E. (1985) Chest physiotherapy in the neonatal intensive care unit. *Physiotherapy.* **71**(2), 63–5.

Pavia D., Thomson M.L. & Clarke S.W. (1978) Enhanced clearance of secretions from the human lung after the administration of hyper-tonic saline aerosol. *American Review of Respiratory Disease.* **117**, 199–203.

Pontoppidan H. (1980) Mechanical aids to lung expansion in non-intubated surgical patients. *American Review of Respiratory Disease.* **122**, suppl. 5(2), 109–19.

Poulton E.P. (1936) Left-sided heart failure with pulmonary oedema. Its treatment with the 'pulmonary plus pressure machine'. *Lancet.* **ii**, 981–3.

Preston I.M., Matthews H.R. & Ready A.R. (1986) Minitracheotomy. *Physiotherapy.* **72**(10) 494–7.

Pryor J.A., Parker R.A. & Webber B.A. (1981) A comparison of mechanical and manual percussion as adjuncts to postural drainage in the treatment of cystic fibrosis in adolescents and adults. *Physiotherapy.* **67**, 140–1.

Pryor J.A. & Webber B.A. (1979) An evaluation of the forced expiration technique as an adjunct to postural drainage. *Physiotherapy.* **65**(10) 304–7.

Pryor J.A., Webber B.A., Hodson M.E. & Batten J.C. (1979) Evaluation of the forced expiration technique as an adjunct to postural drainage in treatment of cystic fibrosis. *British Medical Journal.* **2**, 417–8.

Purcell M. (1976) Response in the newborn to raised upper airway resistance. *Archives of Disease in Childhood.* **51**, 602–7.

Ravitch M.M. (1983) Chest wall deformities 415–39. In *General Thoracic Surgery.* (ed. T.W. Shields 2nd ed.) Lea & Febiger.

Reid L. (1973) Development and anatomy of the lung. *Medicine.* **13**, 811–6.

Rehder K., Hatch D.J., Sessler A.D. & Fowler W.S. (1972) The function of each lung of anesthetized and paralyzed man during mechanical ventilation. *Anesthesiology.* **37**(1), 16–26.

Reiser J. & Warner J.O. (1986) Inhalation treatment for asthma. *Archives of Disease in Childhood.* **61**, 88–94.

Renwick B.M. (1985) Periodic continuous positive airway pressure. *New Zealand Journal of Physiotherapy.* **13**(1), 12–13.

Roberton N.R.C. (1986) *A Manual of Neonatal Intensive Care,* 2nd ed. Edward Arnold, London.

Rosenbluth M. & Chernick V. (1974) Influence of mist tent therapy on sputum viscosity and water content in cystic fibrosis. *Archives of Disease in Childhood.* **49**, 606–10.

Roussos C.S., Fixley M., Genest J. *et al.* (1977) Voluntary factors influencing the distribution of inspired gas. *American Review of Respiratory Disease.* **116**, 457–67.

Ruffin R.E., Fitzgerald J.D. & Rebuck A.S. (1977) A comparison of the bronchodilator activity of Sch 1000 and salbutamol *Journal of Allergy and Clinical Immunology.* **59**, 136–41.

Schoeffel R.E., Anderson S.D. & Altounyan R.E.C. (1981) Bronchial hyperactivity in response to inhalation of ultrasonically nebulised solutions of distilled water and saline. *British Medical Journal.* **283**, 1285–7.

Seal P.V. (1974) Analgesia in the treatment of chest injuries. *Physiotherapy.* **60**(5), 134–7.

Shapiro H.M. (1975) Intracranial hypertension: therapeutic and anesthetic considerations. *Anesthesiology.* **43**(4), 445–71.

Shenfield G.M., Evans M.E. & Paterson J.W. (1974) The effect of different nebulisers with and without intermittent positive pressure breathing on the absorption and metabolism of salbutamol. *British Journal of Clinical Pharmacology.* **1**, 295–300.

Simonds A.K., Parker R.A. & Branthwaite M.A. (1986a) Effects of protriptyline on sleep related disturbances of breathing in restrictive chest wall disease. *Thorax.* **41**, 586–90.

Simonds A.K., Parker R.A. & Branthwaite M.A. (1986b) Intermittent positive pressure hyperinflation (IPPH) in restrictive chest wall disease. *Thorax.* **41**, abstract, 244–5.

Sinha R. & Bergofsky E.H. (1972) Prolonged alteration of lung mechanics in kyphoscoliosis by positive pressure hyperinflation. *American Review of Respiratory Disease.* **106**, 47–57.

Spiro S.G. (1986) The staging of lung cancer. In *Recent Advances in Respiratory Medicine 4* (eds D.C. Flenley & T.L. Petty), 261–75, Churchill Livingstone, Edinburgh.

Starke I.D., Webber B.A. & Branthwaite M.A.

(1979) IPPB and hypercapnia in respiratory failure: the effect of different concentrations of inspired oxygen on arterial blood gas tensions. *Anaesthesia.* **34**, 283–7.

Sutton P.P., Parker R.A., Webber B.A. *et al.* (1983) Assessment of the forced expiration technique, postural drainage and directed coughing in chest physiotherapy. *European Journal of Respiratory Diseases.* **64**, 62–8.

Sykes M.K., McNicol M.W. & Campbell E.J.M. (1976) *Respiratory Failure* 2nd ed p. 142 and p. 153, Blackwell Scientific Publications, Oxford.

Thompson B. (1978) *Asthma and Your Child.* 5th ed. Pegasus Press, Christchurch, New Zealand.

Tudehope D.I. & Bagley C. (1980) Techniques of physiotherapy in intubated babies with respiratory distress syndrome. *Australian Paediatric Journal.* **16**, 226–8.

Turner–Warwick M. (1977) On observing patterns of airflow obstruction in chronic asthma. *British Journal of Diseases of the Chest.* **71**, 73–86.

Ward R.J., Danziger F., Bonica J.J. *et al.* (1966) An evaluation of postoperative respiratory maneuvers. *Surgery, Gynecology and Obstetrics.* **123**, 51–4.

Waterhouse J.C. & Howard P. (1983) Breathlessness and portable oxygen in chronic obstructive airways disease. *Thorax.* **38**, 302–6.

Webb M.S.C., Martin J.A., Cartlidge P.H.T. *et al.* (1985) Chest physiotherapy in acute bronchiolitis. *Archives of Disease in Childhood.* **60**, 1078–9.

Webber B.A., Hofmeyr J.L., Morgan M.D.L. & Hodson M.E. (1986) Effects of postural drainage, incorporating the forced expiration technique on pulmonary function in cystic fibrosis. *British Journal of Diseases of the Chest.* **80**, 353–9.

Webber B.A., Parker R.A., Hofmeyr J.L. & Hodson M.E. (1985) Evaluation of self-percussion during postural drainage using the forced expiration technique. *Physiotherapy Practice.* **1**, 42–5.

Webber B.A., Shenfield, G.M. & Paterson J.W. (1974) A comparison of three different techniques for giving nebulised albuterol to asthmatic patients. *American Review of Respiratory Disease.* **109**, 293–5.

Wolfsdorf J., Swift D.L. & Avery M.E. (1969) Mist therapy reconsidered; an evaluation of the respiratory deposition of labelled water aerosols produced by jet and ultrasonic nebulizers. *Pediatrics.* **43**, 799–808.

Wollmer P., Ursing K., Midgren B. & Eriksson L. (1985) Inefficiency of chest percussion in the physical therapy of chronic bronchitis. *European Journal of Respiratory Diseases.* **66**, 233–9.

Wood R.E., Wanner A., Hirsch J. & Farrell P.M. (1975) Tracheal mucociliary transport in patients with cystic fibrosis and its stimulation by terbutoline. *American Review of Respiratory Disease.* **11**, 733–8.

Woodcock A.A., Gross E.R. & Geddes D.M. (1981) Oxygen relieves breathlessness in 'Pink Puffers'. *Lancet.* **i**, 907–9.

World Health Organization (1961) Definition and diagnosis of pulmonary disease with special reference to chronic bronchitis and emphysema. *WHO Technical Report Series.* **213**, 15.

Young C.S. (1984) Recommended guidelines for suction. *Physiotherapy.* **70**, 106–8.

Zack M.B., Pontoppidan H. & Kazemi H. (1974) The effect of lateral positions on gas exchange in pulmonary disease. *American Review of Respiratory Disease.* **110**, 49–55.

Index